Yoga Therapy for Parkinson's Disease and Multiple Sclerosis

of related interest

Yoga for a Happy Back
A Teacher's Guide to Spinal Health through Yoga Therapy
Rachel Krentzman
Foreword by Aadil Palkhivala
ISBN 978 1 84819 271 3
eISBN 978 0 85701 253 1

Chair Yoga
Seated Exercises for Health and Wellbeing
Edeltraud Rohnfeld
Illustrated by Edeltraud Rohnfeld
ISBN 978 1 84819 078 8
eISBN 978 0 85701 056 8
ISBN 978 1 84819 184 6 (DVD)

Mudras of Yoga
72 Hand Gestures for Healing and Spiritual Growth
Cain Carroll with Revital Carroll
eISBN 978 0 85701 143 5
ISBN 978 1 84819 176 1 (Cards)

The Supreme Art and Science of Raja and Kriya Yoga
The Ultimate Path to Self-Realisation
Stephen Sturgess
Foreword by Dr. David Frawley
ISBN 978 1 84819 261 4
eISBN 978 0 85701 209 8

Qigong for Multiple Sclerosis
Finding Your Feet Again
Nigel Mills
ISBN 978 1 84819 019 1
eISBN 978 0 85701 029 2

Yoga Therapy

FOR PARKINSON'S DISEASE AND MULTIPLE SCLEROSIS

Jean Danford

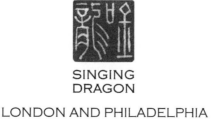

SINGING
DRAGON

LONDON AND PHILADELPHIA

First published in 2016
by Singing Dragon
an imprint of Jessica Kingsley Publishers
73 Collier Street
London N1 9BE, UK
and
400 Market Street, Suite 400
Philadelphia, PA 19106, USA

www.singingdragon.com

Library of Congress Cataloging in Publication Data
Names: Danford, Jean, author.
Title: Yoga therapy for Parkinson's disease and multiple sclerosis / Jean
    Danford.
Description: London ; Philadelphia, PA : Singing Dragon, 2016. | Includes
    bibliographical references and index.
Identifiers: LCCN 2016007636 | ISBN 9781848192997 (alk. paper)
Subjects: | MESH: Parkinson Disease--therapy | Multiple Sclerosis--therapy |
    Yoga
Classification: LCC RC382 | NLM WL 359 | DDC 616.8/330642--dc23 LC record available at
http://lccn.loc.gov/2016007636

British Library Cataloguing in Publication Data
A CIP catalogue record for this book is available from the British Library

ISBN 978 1 84819 299 7
eISBN 978 0 85701 249 4

Printed and bound in Great Britain

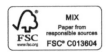

Contents

Disclaimer

This book is meant as a reference guide for yoga teachers and yoga therapists and is not a replacement for medical treatment. If you are concerned for the health of your student, you should advise them to seek medical help. If a student is experiencing pain or pressure in the chest, dizziness, acute pain in the muscles or worsening of symptoms, they should be referred to their doctor immediately.

Acknowledgements

My thanks go to Caroline Evans, specialist Parkinson's nurse, Hereford; Heather Blashki for her kind permission to use her work on hasta mudras; and to all of the students in my specialist classes.

I would also like to thank friends and colleagues who have been patient enough to read through the text, in particular, Carolyn Daniel, Sharon Gisbourne, Alexandra Lyons, Sheila Simmons, Patricia Cronin, Viv Quillin and Richard Booth.

Preface

At a small conference for people with Parkinson's in our local area, all of the health professionals were in unison in promoting exercise as a way of maintaining health and quality of life for people with Parkinson's, and the importance of relaxation and activities to help with stress levels and anxiety. Thus, at my 'stall' I had many visitors asking about yoga. They were eager to join a group and to begin to practise. Alas, my county is huge and mine is the only specialised class, miles away from most of the population. However, most were aware that there may be a yoga class nearby that they could join, and asked me whether that would that work for them. I had to hesitate, knowing the wide range of different types of yoga on offer, and questioning in my mind whether their particular yoga class in the village hall would be okay, whether the teacher would have the skills to adapt postures for them and to understand the condition enough to provide what they need.

I found myself saying 'I would avoid Ashtanga, and Flow classes... Talk to the teacher first. Make sure that your teacher has a good yoga training.' But what does that mean for the average member of the public, when there are so many training schools out there? Many yoga teachers have only done a limited amount of training with very little taught about modifying postures, or even safe practice.

There are many people out there longing to find out what yoga has to offer, and for whom a suitably adapted practice could bring many benefits.

I hope that this book will help yoga teachers to feel that they can teach people with Parkinson's and welcome them into their groups. Many people with Parkinson's avoid classes because they feel embarrassed when they can't manage the posture, or they 'freeze' or shake, and yet with a little tact and sensitivity we can offer a different way and give that person a sense of achievement and belonging with the added benefit of increasing their quality of life. And it is a similar scenario for those with multiple sclerosis (MS).

Chapter 1

My Experience

Quite early in my life I began to see the impact that Parkinson's disease could have on someone's life. First, with an uncle, whose movements were slow and curious to me as a child, but who always looked solemn, and later on, another very dear relative, who, on retiring from a busy and stressful job, was diagnosed with the disease. This changed his sociability, his powers of communication and his enthusiasm for life. I was already into yoga at that time and we discussed how it might help him, and so, encouraged by his wife, he began a daily regime of postures and breathing (Asana and Pranayama). This helped him to stay reasonably mobile and active despite the disease.

So when I was asked to take on a group that had been running for some years for people with Parkinson's disease, I accepted to see what more I could do. This has become an interesting and enjoyable session with lovely caring people, so supportive of one another, and the highlight of my week. They have taught me about the disease, how its symptoms are managed, and how differently it affects people; they have shown me what can and can't be done, and what can be achieved by focus and mental application.

Many years ago I was offered work as a yoga teacher within a psychiatric unit at my local general hospital. Having had little hands-on experience in this area as a specialism, I fell back on my basic yoga training, which fortunately was broad and based on a 'yoga for health' model. I stayed in this post for ten years or more, and learned much. This led me to work with a special needs group at my local college, a group of very mixed students – two were in wheelchairs, others with mental illnesses, and some with limited physical mobility after experiencing road accidents. This gave me experience beyond my official training.

My work with people with multiple sclerosis (MS) has been largely on a one-to-one basis, as each individual can be at a very different stage of the disease, from wheelchair-bound to able-bodied. I was always on the lookout for new ways that I could offer yoga to assist these students, carefully watching them to see how they responded and which approaches worked. I was thirsty for knowledge, and I still am.

I hope that this book will encourage yoga teachers to work with groups like this. Far from being limited and mundane in yoga practice, they are rewarding and inspiring, a fertile learning ground for all involved.

To some, all yoga is therapeutic. It is possible to bring about positive change using a general yoga teaching approach, adapting postures and offering a class that includes breathing and relaxation. A good, inclusive yoga teaching qualification will give a teacher adequate skills to offer this.

My message here is that Yoga Therapy training is extremely useful but would have given only some of the understanding that I have gained through practical, therapeutic experience. But do not dismiss the good that can be done with the basics, common sense, applying Ahimsa (doing no harm) and having a curious and inventive mind.

I added to my yoga teaching skills by studying further, with training in a psychophysical therapy, Postural Integration, which is akin to Rolfing and Emotional Therapy. This reinforced my belief and understanding that body and mind are one, and that working on the physical can bring about transformation in the mental and emotional fields, a belief, for me, supported by the yoga Pancha kosha model. I have developed many of my subtle energy techniques by blending these approaches together. What I knew to be effective in the body-mind model is now being proven and explored as neuroception and interoception, in the field of neuroscience. The outcomes of my work have come not from research (and I am not a medic); they have come from my hands-on experience with people, over many years.

Yoga Therapy helps us to understand the depth of the individual condition. While seeking therapy for one thing – Parkinson's, for example – what is often revealed is another underlying issue. This may be a belief, a state of being, and we may find that this underpins everything else. A karmic pattern may be revealed. We seldom get to this in a group situation, but in one-to-one work there is the opportunity to go below the surface, if the student is ready.

It is easy to get distracted by the need within ourselves as teachers to see measurable improvements. We want to see better balance, improved stability. We want to offer the dream of this condition not getting any worse. But let us not forget the goal of yoga – peace of mind, inner stillness, or even enlightenment.

I sometimes modify these goals with a modern psychotherapeutic approach, 'to be the best I can be, with all my faults, quirks and health conditions' today. It is known that if we can improve breathing, relax and stay mobile, the organism is less likely to fall into a cycle of illness and added health complications.

Both Parkinson's and MS are not going to go away for those with the diagnosis. It may incur fear, anger and despair, and these may continue as the disease process takes away the person's normality. Many come to a place of acceptance – not that other emotions stop (we never stop feeling), but adjustments are made, and building from a new place, a new way of being begins. What does not change is the inner being, and maintaining this connection is what yoga does best.

What is Parkinson's disease?

One person in every 500 has Parkinson's. That's about 127,000 people in the UK.

Most people who get Parkinson's are aged 50 or over but younger people can get it too. (Parkinson's UK)

Parkinson's is a progressive neurological condition, where the cells that produce the chemical dopamine cease to function and die. Dopamine enables nerve messages to be transmitted from the brain to the muscle. Interruption in its flow means that the message doesn't get through properly, causing dysfunction in muscle control and mobility, which sometimes results in the classic Parkinson's symptoms – tremors, a shuffling walk and lack of facial expression. Other symptoms are rigidity, muscle spasm and 'freezing'. People also find that they may suffer from tiredness, pain, depression and constipation. As well as the physical problems caused by motor activity, the area of the brain responsible for motor activity is also responsible for mood, so people with Parkinson's are susceptible to anxiety and may also be depressed. The disease process and the speed of its progression are different for everyone, but these should all be taken into account when planning a yoga programme.

Treatment of Parkinson's disease

There is currently no cure for Parkinson's, and the cause is not known. It is managed by a drug regime, occasionally surgery and other supportive therapies. Drug treatments aim to increase the level of dopamine that reaches the brain, and to stimulate the parts of the brain where dopamine works. There are many different drugs prescribed for Parkinson's, and it is helpful for a yoga therapist to understand how these work, and how they may affect behaviour, muscle control and energy levels.

Levodopa is the main drug treatment for Parkinson's, and in the UK these are Madopar and Sinemet® (it may be prescribed under different names in different countries); the body changes this drug into dopamine. It is important to consider the side effects when looking to plan Yoga Therapy, as the following may be reported:

- confusion

- hallucinations and delusions

- mood swings

- psychological changes

- sleepiness, fainting or dizziness.

If students report these, advise them to refer to their specialist nurse.

There are many other drugs that supplement the activity of dopamine, either damping down the motor responses that cause tremors, by boosting the uptake of dopamine, or slowly releasing dopamine into the system. Deep brain stimulation is being used more frequently for those for whom dyskinesis (severe trembling) is a growing problem during their 'off' times. According to Parkinson's UK:

> In deep brain stimulation signals from an electrical implant in the brain help reduce Parkinson's symptoms, such as tremor and stiffness. Deep brain stimulation is not a cure, but it can give some people better control of their symptoms. It may help to reduce some movement symptoms of Parkinson's, such as slowness of movement, stiffness and tremor. It may also mean that someone has to take less medication, which can reduce the risk of side effects, such as involuntary movements (dyskinesia).

In providing Yoga Therapy, the pacing of the drug regime needs to be considered, as this will affect the optimal time when the student will be active. Parkinson's has daily on/off phases: the terms 'on/off' or 'motor fluctuations' refer to the period when people can no longer rely on the smooth and even symptom control that their drugs once gave them. Each individual will need to consider this, along with the timing of yoga practice.

Exercise is essential for both quality of life and for maintaining mobility for as long as possible. Swimming, walking, stretching and other physical activities are encouraged. In some areas Conductive Education is offered, a system of integrated education and therapy that can help any child or adult with a neurological movement problem (cerebral palsy is the most common condition treated). It is also useful for genetic disorders and for adults with Parkinson's, MS, stroke or acquired brain injury.

Parkinson's UK say that an exercise regime will improve the following:

- walking, sitting down, standing up and turning in bed

- keeping joints flexible and relieving the effects of rigidity

- improving or maintaining muscle strength

- balance training and preventing or managing falls

- pain relief through manual therapy

- maintaining or improving effective breathing.

We can see that yoga can help to meet many of these.

The progress of Parkinson's disease is measured by the Hoehn and Yahr scale, a system commonly used for describing, in broad terms, how Parkinson's symptoms progress and the relative level of disability. It was originally published in 1967 in the journal *Neurology* by Margaret Hoehn and Melvin Yahr, and included stages 1–5. Since then, stage 0 has been added, and stages 1.5 and 2.5 have been proposed and are widely used. The stages are as follows:

- Stage 0: No signs of disease.

- Stage 1: Symptoms on one side only (unilateral).

- Stage 1.5: Symptoms are unilateral and also involve the neck and spine.

- Stage 2: Symptoms are on both sides (bilateral), but there is no impairment of balance.

- Stage 2.5: Mild bilateral symptoms with recovery when the 'pull' test is given (the doctor stands behind the person and asks them to maintain their balance when pulled backwards).

- Stage 3: Balance impairment; mild to moderate disease; physically independent.

- Stage 4: Severe disability, but still able to walk or stand unassisted.

- Stage 5: Needing a wheelchair or bedridden unless assisted.

In a clinical setting, however, a more practical evaluation is used based on everyday activities. This asks questions about speech, swallowing, difficulty using utensils, handwriting, difficulty dressing, falling, 'freezing', walking, turning in bed, etc.

What is multiple sclerosis?

Multiple sclerosis (MS) is a condition of the central nervous system, involving the immune system. More than 100,000 people in the UK have MS. Symptoms usually start in the twenties and thirties, and it affects almost three times as many women as men. It is a lifelong condition, and the cause is not known. As yet there is no cure, but research is progressing fast.

In MS, the immune system begins to attack a substance called myelin, which protects the nerve fibres in the central nervous system. This damages the myelin and strips it off the nerve fibres, either partially or completely, leaving scars known as lesions or plaques.

This damage disrupts messages travelling along the nerve fibres – they can slow down, become distorted, or not get through at all. As well as myelin loss, there can also sometimes be damage to the actual nerve fibres. It is this nerve damage that causes the increase in disability that can occur over time.

As the central nervous system links everything the body does, many different types of symptoms can appear in MS.

There are several different types of MS. Relapsing-remitting MS is the most common and first stage of the illness. It may be, but is not always, followed some years later by secondary progressive MS, where disability gradually increases. Other types are primary progressive MS, which usually affects people from their mid-forties onwards, and does not have the relapse-remission pattern, and benign MS, where there has been an initial illness with recovery and few symptoms following, although this does not mean that it will not develop.

Treatments for MS include disease-modifying drugs that have an immunomodulating effect. These are often interferon-based and are injected. They work with the immune system in various ways, and often have flu-like side effects that may last 48 hours or so. Various drugs are prescribed to help with symptoms such as tremor, sleep difficulties and tiredness.

Physiotherapy, massage and modifications to diet are also recommended, as well as Yoga Therapy.

MS symptoms include numbness, tingling, loss of muscle strength, paralysis, difficulty balancing and walking, and difficulties with both coordination and dexterity. Spasm and stiffness may be present, and there may also be bladder/bowel problems, speech difficulties and overall mental and physical tension.

There are often accompanying emotional disturbances, depression, anxiety, mood swings frustration and fears. Tiredness is a debilitating problem with this disease.

Comparing Parkinson's disease and multiple sclerosis

We can see that both Parkinson's and MS are neurological diseases but have very different causes. Although they affect different age groups, there are similarities in the needs of both groups that can be met through yoga practice. This book may therefore be useful for working with both of these groups as:

- both have mobility and movement issues

- both have spasm, stiffness and balance problems

- in both cases there is disruption to daily life and possible depressive conditions, tiredness, loss of confidence and quality of life.

Cautionary note

As I am not a medical doctor, nor a research scientist, my experience is from directly working with people, and so the practices and methods suggested in this book are to be used alongside orthodox medical treatment, and they should not be used instead of orthodox treatment.

It is always best to refer a student to their specialist nurse or doctor if is there is any doubt as to whether a particular yoga practice would be contraindicated.

How yoga makes a difference

A small survey of our practising groups has shown that for MS, in a range of practices covering joint mobilising, strengthening, stretching, balancing, relaxation, breathing and visualisation, the most helpful, and the one that the students themselves perceived as producing a noticeable beneficial effect, was relaxation, followed by strengthening and breathing practices. All of the students reported feeling energised and well after the sessions. We asked if partners were able to note any differences. Those that reported back commonly said that their partner was calmer, steadier, moving better and sleeping well after yoga practice.

A similar survey of our Parkinson's students over the same practices – joint mobilising, strengthening, stretching, balancing, breathing relaxation and visualisation – found that stretching and joint mobilising were the practices that they enjoyed and found the most useful. Students reported feeling more mobile and energised after class. Although it was hard for them to identify any specific improvements in their condition, they all reported feeling better and generally well, and noticed a difference if they did not attend class. It clearly helped them to maintain useful movement and to stay active, and their partners noticed that they moved better and were calmer after yoga.

Research into the effects of yoga for Parkinson's disease and multiple sclerosis

There have been various studies looking into the impact of yoga on Parkinson's and MS, and I present below some of the more relevant ones in this section.

Parkinson's-related research

Kaitlyn Roland completed her PhD research at the University of British Columbia (2012), which measured Parkinson's disease-related changes to daily muscle activity and the consequences for physical function and frailty. She found that yoga not only improved psychological wellbeing, but also had an effect on the mobility problems experienced by many patients.

Boulgarides *et al.* (2008) researched into the effect of an adaptive yoga programme on mobility, function and outlook in individuals with Parkinson's disease. The background for the research was:

> …that Yoga has been found to be effective in addressing problems of strength, flexibility, balance, gait, anxiety, depression, and concentration. These problems are all present to varying degrees in individuals with Parkinson's Disease (PD). Different forms of exercise and therapy have been found to improve the symptoms related to PD, but no experimental studies have been found exploring the effects of a Yoga program on those symptoms.

Their conclusion was that changes in measures of strength, ROM (range of movement), mobility, gait, balance and psychological health indicate a positive effect of yoga for those with Parkinson's, supporting further study using randomised controlled research design with more subjects.

Multiple sclerosis-related research

The research results of yoga for MS are much more mixed, although several studies have shown that yoga practice relieves fatigue. In early 2008, The Expanding Light yoga school co-sponsored a research study of Ananda yoga that included energisation exercises, a combination of deep breathing, isometric contraction and mental focus to increase body awareness and neuromuscular coordination. The purpose of the study was to investigate the effects of this yoga routine on various aspects of day-to-day functioning and quality of life in individuals with MS. The results of the study showed encouraging positive results on many fronts, including improvements in balance, strength, levels of anxiety and depression, feeling of vitality, concentration and a sense of wellbeing.

The Rutgers School of Health Related Professions recently conducted a pilot trial (see Fogerite *et al.* 2014). Those who participated were better able to walk for short distances and longer periods of time, had better balance while reaching backwards, fine motor coordination, and were better able to go from sitting to standing. Their quality of life also improved in perceived mental health, concentration, bladder control, walking and vision, with a decrease in pain and fatigue.

Almost all of the research projects recommend further research with larger groups for a more accurate picture.

Chapter 2

An Exploration of the Holistic Yoga Approach and How It Can Help

Because on the surface both Parkinson's and MS present in such a physical way, it is hard not to see that making improvements to physical wellbeing is all that is needed to make a huge difference to someone with these diagnoses. And yet yoga, more than any other therapy, is bound up in the concept of what makes up a human being, and what makes that being whole.

Although Western medicine separates out the systems of the body, and seeks to find the origin of the disease process to find a cure, Eastern medicine looks at a much more subtle construct of health and wellbeing, the energy or life force known as prana, which acts as a blueprint for the whole organism. Understanding how that energy flows and manifests as prana vayu to sustain the organism, or becomes stagnant or restricted, forms a different view of ill health.

There are several models that serve as a means of looking at the qualities of each individual and therefore the kind of yoga practices that will be useful. The model of the three gunas (qualities of nature) describes states of inertia, activity or balance. Ayurveda uses the system of doshas to categorise each person and to find the treatment that will best work with their type. Yoga has the principle of Pancha kosha, an overview of the different parts of a human being from the physical to the spiritual, and even more subtle is the chakra system underlying all.

Although I do not go into great detail about all of these systems, we can use them to understand these diseases from a yoga viewpoint, and to help guide the practices that will support the human being into a state of wellness.

Only in the last century have psychologists, and neural scientists, come to see that the emotional, social interactiveness and thought processes of the individual have a great bearing on overall health, stress levels and happiness, and that these influence the body's ability to heal itself.

In the next section we will see what yoga can do, and how the different models can inform therapeutic practice.

Looking after the whole person

When assessing the needs of individuals with a view to setting a yoga practice, for any health problem, the Pancha kosha (maya) model gives us a simple way of observing the person from five different aspects:

- Annamaya kosha, the physical body, supporting the needs of the body, its functions and activities.

- Pranamaya kosha, the energy body. Although we access prana (life force) from other sources (our food, water and environment), focusing on the ability to breath well is vital, as the pranic body provides a 'blueprint' to support the physical systems.

- Manomaya kosha, the mental/emotional body. The lower mental function operates here, including all our emotional ups and downs. Working at this level is key to enhancing wellbeing, and bringing about mental clarity and a calm emotional disposition.

- Vijnanamaya kosha, the wisdom body, engages the intellect and higher faculties of the mind. In this place we see from a different point of view, understand things differently, adapt and learn.

- Anandamaya kosha, often referred to as the 'bliss body', needs to be nourished adequately. In lay terms, this refers to our ability to find contentment and inspiration.

The koshas do not really operate as layers; they are imprinted into the fabric of our being and work together to form the whole. They are interdependent.

In people with limited mobility, one would think that the physical level is the one demanding most attention, but this is not the case. Practices that support and balance the emotional and mental faculties will have just as much, if not more, benefit to the overall health and wellbeing of the person.

Some examples of practices and activities that can nourish and balance each kosha level are shown below.

How we might support and balance the koshas

Annamaya kosha, the physical body

Asana, mobility, stability and awareness

It has been shown that exercise is paramount for people with Parkinson's. Rather than being limited by the disease, staying active and working the body keeps people active and independent for longer, giving a better quality of life and enabling people to engage in normal, everyday life for much longer than was previously thought possible. In people with MS, mobility, strength and stability are important in combating the effects of the disease. Yoga is excellent in that it is easily adaptable and can offer a variety of useful practices. Asanas have a positive effect throughout all of the systems of the body as well as on the musculoskeletal system. Asana practice improves digestion, elimination, heart and lung function, and impacts the brain, nervous and endocrine activity in a positive way.

Firmly in the field of Annamaya, in relation to the physical body for people with Parkinson's is the issue of posture, which often becomes stooped, or Pisa syndrome can develop, where the person leans to one side. A study by Dr Karen Doherty *et al.* (2013) said that:

> While most of the people who took part in our study had difficulty correcting their posture by themselves, few actually had permanent changes in their spine… The changes we saw tended to involve muscles and joints becoming stuck in the wrong position – like bent knees or a tilted pelvis. This suggests that people may benefit from non-surgical interventions like physiotherapy.

In MS the issue may be more one of steadiness and balance.

In yoga, asana practice can go a long way in helping towards better posture and increased awareness to help strengthen the core muscles, proprioception and balance, thus avoiding the aches and pains that come with poor posture.

There are other therapies that may help. It is acknowledged that some complementary therapies are helpful for Parkinson's – aromatherapy, reflexology, massage, chiropractic, osteopathy and physiotherapy, Conductive Education, as well as walking and swimming are all ways of staying active and stimulated.

Supporting Annamaya with diet
The digestive system in both Parkinson's and MS can become sluggish as the muscular action of the gut is affected, which can cause poor absorption and constipation. Moving and stretching can help with this.

Diet and Parkinson's
Proteins can interfere with the way Levodopa is used by the body, so it is essential that dietary recommendations are followed, at the same time getting all the nutritional elements needed for health. The Parkinson's UK booklet on diet refers to research where people reduced the amount of daytime protein they ate to improve their response to Levodopa, which can help some people. A protein redistribution diet is sometimes suggested where most protein is eaten in the evening.

It is important, however, to keep eating protein as it is an essential part of nutrition, and is vital to help the body to renew itself and fight infection. Reducing protein may cause dangerous weight loss. Following general guidelines for keeping weight steady, eating plenty of fibre, fruit and vegetables, and drinking adequate amounts of water are all advised.

Diet and multiple sclerosis

According to the MS Trust:

> Whether it is possible to influence multiple sclerosis through diet and dietary supplements is a controversial topic. There is much information available in books, magazines and on the web, much of it contradictory. Opinions range from denying any evidence of benefit to suggesting that MS can effectively be cured by particular diets.

It goes on to suggest that, for many people with MS, managing what they eat offers the possibility of a sense of control in dealing with their condition. Poor diet and nutrition can also worsen existing symptoms such as fatigue and weakness. Awareness of diet also offers the opportunity to promote general health and wellbeing, which may be even more important following a diagnosis of MS.

It seems that fats and vitamin D have a part to play, although it remains a controversial subject, with many conflicting views and research, but exploring for yourself what diet works best for you would be an important way of supporting Annamaya.

Pranamaya kosha, the energy body

Breathing exercises and Pranayama

If there is no energy to draw on, we get pulled into a negative spiral: no energy – no motivation – begin to feel weak – can't engage in activity – feel self-conscious and lack confidence – life becomes limited and the whole cycle starts again. If the lungs aren't functioning well, nor is the heart or the circulation, and we become even more depleted in energy. Breathing practices not only bring improvement to the health of these organs but will also lift overall energy levels and improve mental outlook. However physically limited one might be, working with the breath is always possible.

Other activities such as singing are helpful to focus on controlling the breath and to keep lungs healthy.

Manomaya kosha, the mental body

Mind/emotions: deep relaxation, Pratyahara, yoga nidra, visualisation, affirmation, and meditation help in staying positive and keeping calm

A diagnosis of Parkinson's or MS may bring with it depression. Feelings of helplessness, hopelessness and low self-worth may follow. Meditation practices can begin to re-set expectations and bring a quality of aliveness that is felt when we 'live in the moment'. At this level of being we are able to use yoga practices to find balance, and to move towards positive thinking and deal with negative thoughts and fears.

Anxiety is commonly found in people with Parkinson's and MS, and yoga offers many practices to change this; breathing, relaxation and meditation can all help to re-balance the nervous system and implement positive changes.

If you are working one-to-one, you may be able to provide a resource by just listening. When the medical regime presents problems, and medication is not working as expected, people with Parkinson's will often feel angry and frustrated. These are feelings that may spill over into their family circle, or that they want to hide from the people who care for them, in order not to burden them further. At such times, someone outside of their caring team who has no other involvement may be those to whom it is safe to express these emotions – expression is healthier than repression.

Vijnanamaya kosha, the wisdom body

Wisdom and function of the higher mind and intellect

When we are open to learning, and able to reflect on life, lessons are learned and positive changes can be made. We might find inspiration in many places. When life brings challenges, we have an opportunity to review what works and what doesn't. Day-to-day living itself will be a challenge for many with Parkinson's or neurological problems, but if we remove the filters of fear and depression, there may be many helpful things to learn. In the yoga tradition many would turn to the ancient texts of the Bhagavad Gita and Patanjali's Sutras for guidance. There are equivalents in other traditions, but it may be that we are inspired by friends, health workers, classmates, internet forums, educational films as well as many other sources.

Keeping an open mind is essential.

Anandamaya kosha, the 'bliss body'

Finding inspiration, remembering to play, finding the ah! moments

Connecting with a part of yourself that takes you into a different realm, where you can experience spiritual connection and upliftment, is profound and beautiful. Rather than stumbling across these moments, we can actively seek them. Finding beauty and awe links us to a part of our being that is fulfilling like no other. Watch the sea, see the sunset, look at the stars, sit in a cathedral – lift out of the everyday.

It is essential that first and foremost we offer yoga within the guidance of Patanjali and Ahimsa (non-violence), working with compassion and understanding.

How Patanjali's Sutras guide the therapeutic approach

Patanjali's Sutras offer an underpinning of philosophy for therapeutic yoga. In *Sutra 1.2, Chitta vrtti nirodhah*, restraint of the modifications of the mind, Patanjali infers that the unadulterated mind state is pure and clear. Our thoughts – all of them – are disturbances. To bring them into a peaceful state is a challenge for even the healthiest individual. How much more challenging then when Parkinson's or MS is diagnosed.

Even the word 'yoga' has a definition of unity, and implies balance, harmonising the body and mind, inner and outer. Yoga is all about changing the world within, bringing new perspectives. Rather than enlightenment being a saintly state of bliss, we can gain some kind of liberation by freeing ourselves from fear and limitations imposed by our own thinking and beliefs. Reconnecting with the true self, and understanding who, how and what that is brings a very different viewpoint of life, one that is not conditional on the physical state. And when we are in balance, follow *Sutra 1.3, Tada drasthu svarupe vasthanam*, then the self/seer abides in its own nature. This leads to self-realisation.

However, we are not in a calm, balanced, clear place most of the time. We are pulled and pushed by the activities of the mind and in a reactive state of being. Patanjali goes on to describe these modifications, the vrtti, some of which bring suffering and some joy. In order to find balance, Patanjali urges practice. With these Sutras in mind, we can see that when illness is chronic and prolonged, more determination is needed to overcome distractions.

Distractions are listed in *Sutra 1.30* – they are obstacles to progress. *Vyahhi styana samshaya pramada alasya avirati bhranti-darshana alabdha-bhumikatva anavasthitatva chitta vikshepa te antarayah* – vyahhi, disease is the first obstacle, followed by dullness, carelessness, laziness, sensuality, false perception, failure to reach firm ground, and slipping back from progress made, complete the list.

In *Sutra 1.31, duhkha daurmanasya angam-ejayatva shvasa prashvasah vikshepa sahabhuva*, distress, despair, trembling of the body and disturbed breathing are identified.

All of these would be easily identifiable in a person with Parkinson's or MS. The disease can overtake life completely so that the idea of a true self existing and being able to connect with that part is left far behind. Although there is desire to ease or even overcome some of the physical symptoms of the disease, there is also a need for the individual to be preserved and not lost in the disease process. Woven into yoga sessions should be the underpinning philosophy that the self dwells within and can be nurtured, recognised and present. Thus the quality of life is enhanced.

Patanjali goes on to say that focused practice is the best way to overcome distractions. Perseverance, practice and focus can all be encouraged within the yoga practices planned. We need to motivate, encourage, educate and inform, so that students feel supported in moving forward. It is in this area that we can offer practice sheets, describing 10–20 minute sessions to be done at home, to engage regular practice.

In *Sutra 1.33, Maitri karuna mudita upekshanam sukha duhka punya apunya vishayanam bhavanatah chitta prasadanam*, Patanjali states that by being friendly and compassionate and not focusing on the negatives, the mind is able to become calm.

In recent years we have seen studies in the field of neurophysiology that show that these attitudes help in healing stress and trauma, the part of the nervous system responsive to the social environment and relationships. The vagus nerve and the enteric nervous system respond to friendliness, compassion, warmth and love, which bring about positive changes in health, and the human being can move towards homeostasis (Porges 2011).

It is important to encourage this attitude both as a leader of a group and among the group members themselves. My observation in working with small groups, especially those connected to a charitable network where there is social interaction as well as education, is that by care, consideration and inclusiveness, one can bring about a sense of belonging and wellbeing that supports the progress made in other areas of yoga practice.

Patanjali goes on to offer breathing, awareness/mindfulness and meditation as practices that lessen the power of negative, hurtful, traumatic memories and experiences, and lead to a better quality of life.

In the second part of Patanjali's Sutras, 2.3–9, the five obstacles – kleshas – are described, and we are reminded that they are ever-present. These are ignorance, egoism, attachment, hatred and clinging to bodily life. Ignorance in this instance is not just a lack of knowledge or education, but not being able to see the truth. When we are caught up in suffering, our ability to recognise what is real diminishes.

Do our students want to engage in this search for the truth? As with yoga itself, and in life in general, some people are drawn to be seekers and others follow a different path. If this concept is at the heart of our teaching, I believe the quality and vibration of that message will get through. In many people, illness causes introspection and leads them to question the things in life of real value, to prioritise differently, to value life experiences differently. This, in its essence, is therapeutic.

As yoga teachers, we are encouraged to offer a spread of practices following the guidelines set by Patanjali, known commonly as 'The Eight Limbs of Yoga': Yama, Niyama, Asana, Pranayama, Prtyahara, Dharana, Dhyana and Samadhi. In planning a balanced yoga session, these offer a framework of underpinning ethics, moral standpoint, practices and progression.

Patanjali's 'Eight Limbs' offer the model defining yoga practice in working towards the goal of a healthy contented life.

Yama and Niyama underpin our teaching and guide our conduct and attitudes.

Yama is usually translated as restraints, which govern our conduct towards both ourselves and towards others:

- Ahimsa is the refusal of violence, or non-harming.

- Asteya is the refusal of stealing.

- Aparigraha is the refusal of covetousness.

- Satya is truthfulness.

- Brahmacharya is continence.

This group of rules guides us to respect and honour ourselves and others, to show our acknowledgment that there is a oneness in life, doing unto others as you would have done to yourself.

Niyama translates as observances:

- Saucha is purity.

- Tapas is austerity.

- Samtosa is contentment.

- Svadhyaya is self-study.

- Isvara pranidhana is devotion to the divine.

This group of rules offers guidance on how to conduct oneself and one's thoughts to promote balance and happiness.

Asana offers a range of postures that are specifically tailored to the needs of the student and their capabilities. In asana practice we can improve balance, strengthen muscles and joint mobility, improve circulation and build overall confidence.

Pranayama offers suitable practices that improve oxygen intake and the efficiency and health of the lungs, thus keeping away infections.

Pratyahara is a key practice in aiding physical relaxation and offering an opportunity for inner awareness and inner stillness, bringing an experience of the self, with senses withdrawn.

Dharana offers training to focus concentration and to make progress towards meditation, which is helpful in daily living as we engage the nervous system and brain function.

Dyana is meditation. Although there may not be an opportunity to offer this as a practice within the time allowed in a Yoga Therapy group, students can be encouraged to go to a specialist practice group or to practise at home.

Samadhi is a personal experience that would be beyond the remit of the average therapy class.

Guidance for dealing with negative thinking is given in 2.33 and 2.34. When negative thoughts are troubling, think the opposite way – Pratipaksha Bhavana. We can engage with this in therapeutic yoga by offering positive ideas and thinking even in a small way.

Parkinson's disease, multiple sclerosis and the chakra system

There is a point of view that the pranic flow is the origin of health, and when that flow becomes disturbed, ill health follows. The disturbance of energy may begin long before the disease is identified. Many yoga teachers are familiar with the subtle energy system of the chakras, and if we consider what is happening at the subtle energy level, we can see the way that Parkinson's disease and similarly MS show energy imbalance.

The chakras are distribution centres, sending energy out to all the different kosha (levels), through the nervous system, endocrine system and organs of the body, giving us a 3D model. In yoga terminology this happens through the nadis and vayus. We can see how this would impact on the functioning of the whole if it is out of balance.

Just how disturbance manifests in Parkinson's or MS is summarised over the next few pages. This is a projected general analysis as each individual has their own unique pattern.

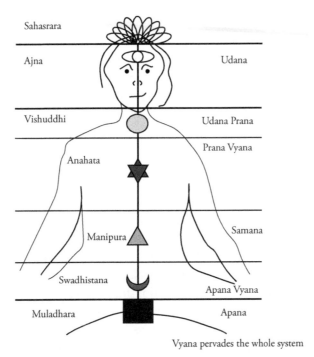

Sahasrara

Ajna · Udana

Vishuddhi · Udana Prana

Prana Vyana

Anahata

Manipura · Samana

Swadhistana

Apana Vyana

Muladhara · Apana

Vyana pervades the whole system

The Chakra and Prana Vayu
showing how they relate to the physical body

The root chakra: Muladhara

What we can observe in Parkinson's and MS is that communication between the brain and body is not functioning. As this affects mobility and ability to control movements, we can expect a severe disruption in Muladhara chakra. So we have instability, loss of balance and disrupted function of walking. Postures can be offered to stabilise, strengthen and energise Muladhara. It is unlikely that there would be a permanent change. It has to be worked regularly to improve quality of life.

On an emotional level, there will be a degree of fear held here that will block energy flow, fear of falling and fear of the condition itself.

The sacral chakra: Swadhisthana

Dopamine is responsible for the experience of pleasure as well as being vital in transmitting messages to the muscles. It is here in Swadhisthana that we find the link into 'desire'; this can be over-stimulated by the medication treating Parkinson's. It can result in out-of-balance behaviour, or over-spending and seeking out pleasurable stimulation as desires intensify (medication is needed to keep this in balance).

As this centre is also to do with power, issues around loss of power will deplete the sacral centre. This may show in MS as mobility is affected and people with MS may become more reliant on others.

Freeing up the lower back, pelvis and hips can help keep the energy flowing.

The solar plexus chakra: Manipura

This is the chakra associated with self-confidence and being comfortable with our own identity as well as linking with the process of digestion. A diagnosis of Parkinson's or MS can really knock self-esteem and self-confidence; there is a loss of sense of self and it is difficult to 'digest' the new situation. It is important when teaching to keep language positive and upbeat, giving encouragement and building week by week, encouraging the class to stay active, to mark achievements and to set goals that are achievable.

The heart chakra: Anahata

Although the Anahata chakra governs the physical heart and the function of respiration, it is here that we really engage with our emotions and where fear can block the energy flow – fear of the future, fear of losing oneself, losing touch with the true self, anxiety for just the everyday activities that become harder. As people become more dependent on others, relationships are tested. All of this will impact on Anahata. We may also lose love for ourselves, not liking what we are becoming.

The heart centre is linked to the thymus, a major organ of the immune system; this may be significant for MS, as it is a disease of the immune system.

The throat chakra: Vishuddhi

The throat is a command centre, governing to some extent the chakras below it. It is the centre of communication, governing speech and the voice.

In Parkinson's the voice is often affected as the muscles weaken. People with Parkinson's may not be able to vocalise their feelings, may be unable to express themselves, or may feel shame about their condition. Using the voice is both empowering and strengthening. Mantras may be useful in energising this centre, or singing, if a mantra is not appropriate – both will also ease and exercise the lungs. Using laughter to encourage is also helpful.

The brow chakra: Ajna

If we look at the physical aspects of this centre, we can see that it is here that the Parkinson's malfunction originates – cells in the brain being unable to produce dopamine. So we have a disruption of the energy of Ajna. Ajna governs mental faculty, so here, again, we see loss of control. The brain is still able to function, but in some cases there is loss affecting memory and communication with other parts of the body, as motor function is lost.

In modern terms, we are told that it is possible to retrain our memory patterns, our nerve functions, owing to the plasticity of the brain. Understanding in this field is in the early days, but yoga provides a great opportunity to work the body/brain connection.

The crown chakra: Sahasrara

This is usually thought of as our spiritual connection. Each person often has a very personal experience of their own spiritual connection, and mostly this subject is outside of the remit of an hour-long class.

We cannot know each individual viewpoint without a deep conversation, but there are some difficulties in upholding a meditative practice. Disease, dullness, carelessness, laziness, false perception, failure to establish the practice, physical unsteadiness, distress, despair and disturbed breathing, these are all are obstacles to progress, as detailed by Patanjali in 1.30–31. However, if there is consistent application towards opening at this level, who knows what may be achieved?

Practices for working on the chakras can be found on pages 246–256.

The five vayus (the five movements or functions of prana)

From the yogic point of view the body is a collection of energy channels. The vayus describe physical flow and function within the systems of the body. This is seen in digestion and elimination, circulation of the blood, the electrical and chemical communication of the nervous system and the action of breathing. The biological workings of the body, its maintenance and repair, its constructive and destructive processes are directed by vayu. Vayu is the cosmic life force or bio energy that creates these channels.

We have five types of prana in the body: prana, apana, vyana, udana and samana.

- Prana vayu flow is inwards and upward. It nourishes the brain and the eyes and governs reception of all things: food, air, senses and thoughts. This is the fundamental energy in the body, and directs and feeds into the four other vayus. Inhaling is the most obvious action of prana.

- Apana vayu energy pervades the lower abdomen. The flow of apana vayu is downwards and out, and its energy nourishes the organs of digestion, reproduction and elimination. Apana vayu governs the elimination of all substances from the body: carbon monoxide, urine, stools, etc.

- Vyana vayu is situated in the heart and lungs and flows throughout the entire body. The flow of vyana vayu moves from inside to outside. It governs the circulation of all substances throughout the body, and assists the other vayus with their functions. We see its action in the circulation of blood and the peripheral nervous system.

- Udana vayu has a circular flow around the neck and head. It functions to 'hold us up' and governs speech, self-expression and growth.

- Samana vayu is situated in the abdomen with its energy centred in the navel. The flow of samana vayu moves from outside to inside. It governs the digestion and assimilation of all substances: food, air, experiences, emotions and thoughts.

In any diseased state these energies are out of balance, and the life force is not flowing. Yoga asana seeks to bring balance and flow in these vital forces. Prana and apana are the major forces, prana supporting and sustaining life and therefore supporting all of the others, and apana, energy leaving the body, is also essential for health. If apana is not flowing effectively, we suffer from congestive conditions, poor breathing, sluggish digestion, constipation and low-energy states.

Because of the individuality of the disease process, the effect on the vayu may be seen differently in each person. In general, in Parkinson's one would assume that udana, the upward-moving energy, supporting thinking and the brain, speech and self-expression, would be depleted. But as in any illness it is best to work on balancing the whole and to strengthen the whole, rather than focusing on just one element.

Yoga Therapy

There are many different ways to deliver Yoga Therapy, and some will work in a traditional way that will include Ayurveda treatments. As it takes many years to train in Ayurveda medicine, the methods of Yoga Therapy offered here seek to bring improvement in the health and wellbeing of people with MS and Parkinson's for their common symptoms and to improve their quality of life, without the specialist Ayurvedic approach.

Yoga Therapy is at its most effective when it is tailored for each individual. A student's needs may vary, as there may be multiple health issues that need to be taken into consideration in planning practices. Even when working with a small 'therapy' group, each individual must be evaluated and considered, and contraindications for the individual taken into account. Before enrolling anyone into a specialist class, it is essential to take a full medical history. With both Parkinson's and MS, people often reach a stage of immobility and may not be able to attend a class that includes asana. Working one-to-one is more suitable for these people, and breathing, meditation and working with the body, even in a small way, may contribute to that person's quality of life.

The case for creative experimental modification of asana

When building a therapeutic practice, there should be considerations for the actions that we wish to implement. For example, postures that stretch the front of the body are often cited as being beneficial for ailments of the digestive tract. I have seen the Wheel Pose (Upward Bow, Chakrasana), Bow Pose (Dhanurasana) and Dynamic Bow Pose quoted as beneficial for diabetes, and the internet is full of 'this practice is beneficial for this ailment'. If we are working with vulnerable people, we need to exert caution and begin to question 'why?' Many postures are for adepts, which would take many years of practice to accomplish. Students and people coming for Yoga Therapy are not adepts; they are often weak, immobile and ill. So we have to find ways of applying the therapeutic principle, and adapting the asana so that the therapeutic action can be applied.

We may be looking for optimising mobility or building strength and stamina, stretching muscles, improving alignment and posture, relaxing and relieving physical tension, relieving stress, and improving the internal functions.

Although in this book there are many ideas for modifying practices for these particular student groups, in reality your students will be the ones to teach you how to help them. Only they can say where their pain is, what their limitations are, and what other problems they have that need to be taken into account.

Chapter 3

Therapeutic Practices

In this chapter we explore a range of yoga practices suitable for people with Parkinson's or MS or people with limited mobility for other reasons. Many of the postures described will be familiar to yoga teachers, but are offered in easy stages and in simplified and adapted versions, so that even the most physically challenged person can advance. Instructions are given to help the teacher, and points for directing the practice are included.

All of the information for contraindications and safe practice, along with guidelines for good alignment in postures that are familiar to most yoga teachers, will apply to these specialist groups. When working with any group in a therapeutic context, it is essential to have a full picture of each individual's health profile, as this will determine any contraindications for them personally, and will enable you, the teacher, to adapt postures for them.

Planning yoga for Parkinson's disease and multiple sclerosis

When working with these diseases, it is important to consider:

- Evaluating the needs of the individual. People often have other health problems that need to be identified and taken into consideration.

- MS and Parkinson's can also affect the internal muscles as well as the external muscles, so there may be digestive/bowel and bladder issues as well as mobility issues.

- Disempowerment, lack of confidence, low self-esteem, anxiety and depression are often present.

- Low energy states and sleep issues.

- Mobility and the ability to control physical movements may be limited.

- Hands-on help and adjustments, with permission, can make all the difference.

The Pancha kosha model needs to be examined for each individual.

Useful yoga tools are:

- warm-ups and mobilising techniques

- balance practices

- developing awareness – proprioception

- visualisation – bhavana for positive thinking and renewal

- strengthening postures adapted for the individual

- work that helps to ease any muscle spasm, gentle stretches and relaxation

- coordination practices

- relaxation – Pratyahara

- breathing and meditation

- adapting postures with the use of props, to assist the individual.

Considerations in planning for one-to-one or group work

Practicalities

- Class size – can you manage the group safely and give individual attention? (A maximum of 6–8 is recommended.)

- Room size – it should be big enough to accommodate a full class as well as equipment.

- Room temperature – warm but not too hot; check the recommendations for the condition.

- Disabled access to hall/bathroom, etc. Are stairs/lift manageable?

- Chairs – stable/sturdy chairs that will not slide around easily and can be placed on a mat.

- Props – blocks/straps/extra chairs.

- Adaptions for wheelchairs – if the user's feet don't reach the floor, for example.

What you might do with your class

- Assess their stamina – they may tire quickly, so plan for rests.

- If the session is an hour, for MS and Parkinson's allow a maximum time of 20–30 minutes for postures, depending on how people are on the day.

- Warm-ups are essential – work the small joints, fingers and toes, as these become more important in limited mobility issues.

- Give instructions at a suitable speed – don't rush, as there might be cognitive issues.

- Include movements that open the chest, strengthen and stretch. Include plenty of breathing and breath awareness.

- Don't hold poses too long – this may tire them too quickly, and exacerbate spasticity and cramping in the muscles.

- Hands-on adjustments can be gentle but firm, without 'manhandling' forcefully.

The practices are grouped according to their action and benefits to the body for this particular student group; adaptations and modifications are described, and a separate section for chair work is included for ease of reference. Some postures are shown in several places, according to their application.

- Preliminaries and warm-ups
- Asana for:
  ○ posture and the spine
  ○ stability and strength
  ○ shoulders and the upper back
  ○ hips and pelvis
  ○ balance
  ○ superstretches
  ○ restorative postures
  ○ digestion
- Pranayama (breathing) exercises
- Practices for mind and emotions:
  ○ relaxation
  ○ moving into positivity – bhavana, visualisation, affirmations
  ○ meditation
- Chakra practices

Safety and the environment

Before beginning to work with an individual or a small group, there are practicalities and safety aspects to consider:

- Working one-to-one is of great benefit, as full attention can then be given to all aspects of the individual, to their health and wellbeing. However, a great deal of benefit can be gained from working with a small group, as this allows time for giving personal attention and making adjustments, and for teachers to be assured that they can observe everyone in the group.

- Over 6–8 students, it is better for there to be a yoga teacher assistant as well as the main tutor, as help will be needed in giving personal guidance and adjustments. Up to 12 people could be taught together. Alternatively, helpers may be willing to be on hand (but bear in mind that although helpers are willing, they may not have the skills that a trained teacher-therapist has).

- It may be necessary to use touch, to guide the postures and movements that you teach, so be sure to ask permission first before you get 'hands on'.

- The room should be warm but not overheated for those with Parkinson's, but students with MS like a cooler room, as too much heat can be a bother for them. As always with yoga, quietness and time free from interruptions is essential. These groups need all the teacher's attention, so the fewer distractions the better. The floor should be clean and non-slip.

Equipment

- yoga mat
- a stable chair
- blocks, hard and soft
- belt
- resistance band
- blanket
- bolsters are useful for specific practices, but not essential overall.

When setting up, make sure that the chair is placed on a mat so that it can't slip away, and that other support equipment is to hand.

Check that there are no obstacles around the floor. Cables, mats and so on are a hazard, especially for those for whom walking is a challenge.

Points for teachers

The range of ability, mobility, strength and presence of symptoms in both Parkinson's and MS will vary greatly. Even with the same medical diagnosis, each person's experience of the disease process is different, and each person manifests it differently, even though the symptoms look similar. Parkinson's disease does sometimes manifest in younger people, but mostly those with Parkinson's are over 50, and the ageing body needs to be respected. People coming into a yoga class with a Parkinson's diagnosis may have other conditions that need to be taken into account, and many come into class having no experience of yoga before.

Some people are very able and can easily get up and down off the floor, and others cannot do this at all. A preliminary health questionnaire is useful in determining the level of fitness in the group. A range of questions about movement, flexibility and Parkinson's symptoms, along with information on any other medical condition that exists alongside the Parkinson's or MS, give a fuller picture to enable planning a therapeutic programme.

In those with Parkinson's, facial muscles are often severely affected, which means that they may be unable to respond and communicate through facial expression. This can present a challenge for some teachers. As human beings, we communicate meaning and emotions through facial expressions and gestures, and we look for responses from others, which helps us to consider our response. When working with people with Parkinson's, remember that there may not be such a response, and yet personality and intelligence are still present.

In yoga philosophy we have the idea that the atman is eternal and dwells within – the person standing before you is present and engaged; they just can't show it. Speak to the true self element of the person.

It is essential to observe the group each time, before starting, to ascertain if everyone feels well, or whether there are other factors to consider. The timing of medication plays a big part in life for those with Parkinson's, so beginning class before the medication activates can be problematic. People have 'off' days and may have other health issues, so be ready to change your plans.

Key teaching skills and qualities are:

- observation

- modification, adjustments and adaptation of yoga postures and practices

- Ahimsa, working within a non-harming rule

- compassion and respect

- patience.

When teaching a Parkinson's-focused group we need to consider which yoga practices will be of most value. Those that develop the following are more important than 'achieving' a perfect posture. This would be similar in other conditions such as MS and other neurological problems where coordination and muscle strength are affected:

- awareness

- breath

- coordination

- proprioception, balance and stability

- empowerment and self-confidence

- mobility, particularly in the small joints

- strength.

Where there is restriction in the body, there is often a negative dialogue. Here the student is subject to mind chatter of a critical nature, where we have a thought process of 'I can't do this, my body won't respond', 'this hurts', 'I'm too stiff', 'I never get this right'.

This flow needs to be converted into positive optimistic encouragement. Offer some positive phrases, such as 'with each move I release a little more', 'I am feeling looser and freer', 'my muscles are softening and lengthening'.

We can add visualisation, such as 'imagine the muscles releasing and lengthening', 'see them strong and elastic', 'imagine breathing golden light into the stretch', 'imagine pouring golden light into the joint like magical lubricating fluid'.

KEEPING AND IMPROVING THE ABILITY TO 'TRANSFER'

Moving from a chair to the floor and from floor to sitting and standing are all essential skills for life, and it is important to maintain the strength and coordination to do this. Yoga postures practised regularly will give confidence in performing these familiar actions, and the ability to transfer will impact on how the yoga session can flow.

■ Moving from standing to sitting on the floor

Instruction

1. Using a stable chair, stand in front of the chair and place your hands on the seat. Hinge at the hip, and bend both knees.

2. Lower one knee to the ground, steadying yourself with the your hands on the chair.

3. Come down onto all fours, and push the chair away.

4. Lower yourself onto one hip, and then lower yourself down so that you are lying on your side.

5. Roll over onto your back.

◾ Getting up from the floor

Instruction

1. Make sure there is a chair nearby. Crawl over to the chair if need be.

2. Or, from lying, roll onto your side.

3. With one arm, push up so that you are sitting on one hip, legs to the side.

4. Turn onto all fours.

5. Bring one foot forward, and hold the chair for support.

6. Come onto your other foot, and with both knees bent, push up to stand.

◾ Getting up from a chair

Getting up and down out of a chair is something that we all need to work on as we get older, so that we can build and maintain strength.

Instruction

1. Sit in a chair. Practise using the pelvic floor and abdominal muscles. (This is emphasised throughout the book in almost all of the practices as it is an essential factor in stability, mobility and back care.)

2. Keep your feet parallel, and feel them on the floor.

3. Press them into the floor, breathe out and engage the core.

4. Lean forward, keeping the natural curve in the spine, and guide the knees over the toes, reach the arms forward, letting the crown of the head lead the movement.

5. Follow the movement through, lifting off the chair just a few inches, and hold.

6. Try to sit down slowly and control the action. The chair *is* still there.

7. Practise this often.

This exercise can be a challenge for the quadriceps, but practice will improve stability.

◾ Plank Pose (Phalakasana)

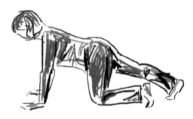 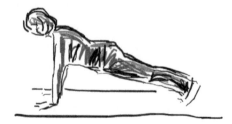

Being able to support our bodyweight is vital in enabling transition out of the chair, and up and down from the floor. This asana can help to maintain that strength and ability. Plank Pose should be worked towards in stages, and progress as the students get stronger.

Instruction

1. Begin with simple weight-bearing poses, such as Cat Pose (see p.50). With the hands and knees placed in correct alignment, transfer the weight of the body forward so that the hands, arms and shoulders bear more weight. This will enable you to get used to taking weight onto the hands, and will help when transferring from lying to sitting to standing.

2. Rock the weight back into the knees, and then repeat the action a few times more. Keep the spine in a straight horizontal line.

3. Breathe in, breathe out, and draw the abdominal muscles in and the pelvic floor up.

4. Lift the knees a little way off the floor, and try to hold.

5. Repeat four times.

Over the weeks, when strength is building, you can progress to:

6. Take one foot back, toes curled under, keeping the hips low and the core muscles engaged.

7. Take the other foot back, taking the weight of the body for a short time, before placing the knees back on the floor.

8. Rest back into your heels with arms stretched forward, in Swan Pose (see page 109).

Progress to full Plank Pose:

9. Keep the hips low and the legs and spine aligned.

■ Side lifts

Instruction

1. Sit on the floor with your legs to the right, and use your left arm as a prop.

2. Engage the pelvic floor.

3. Lift your hips off the floor, taking your weight onto your knees and hand. Come up just as far as you can.

4. Lower yourself back to the floor.

5. Lift and lower four times.

6. Repeat on the other side.

Other useful postures for building strength are:

- Cat balances (see pages 52 and 147) and standing balances (see pages 140–146).

- Chair Pose (Utkatasana) (see page 88).

- Downward-facing Dog Pose (Adho Mukha Svanasana) (see page 106).

Practise these in class regularly. Semi-squat, Cat Pose, leg and arm strengthening will all help to enable these vital movements.

WARM-UPS

It is essential to offer loosening, stretching and mobilising warm-ups before full practice. This will enable you to see how everyone is, to let them become aware of their bodies and begin to focus on what they want out of the session. As with any yoga class, it is good to offer awareness and centring practices and to modify them according to group needs, time of year, temperature and the general demeanour of the group as a whole.

You might offer a standing, sitting or lying start, and you will probably find that there is a mixed range of ability in the group, with some people sitting and some standing. Offering a variety over the weeks means that there is always something that everyone can do as part of the programme.

■ Breath awareness, as a starting focus

This can be done in any position, and allows the student to explore their normal breathing pattern. It can be guided by asking the following:

- Where do you feel your breath?

- Is it low down in your belly, or higher in your chest?

- Can you feel movement in your sides as you breathe?

- Can you feel any movement in your back? Whereabouts in your back can you feel it?

- Where do you feel your breathing starts?

- Can you take your breath down lower?

At this point we have the opportunity to explain full breathing and its benefits, and to follow this with teaching full three-part breath with the focus on experiencing the breath in the front, sides and back of the body.

Parkinson's/MS note: If there is severe curvature of the spine or poor posture, as we often see in Parkinson's, this will limit breathing. Muscle spasm can also be a limiting factor. However, encouraging even the smallest change can be energy-enhancing. Good breathing will have a knock-on effect in the prevention of infections and other breathing problems that can be a complication for people with Parkinson's and MS. Further Pranayama (breathing) practices are discussed in a later section (see page 211). In order to breathe well, the whole musculature needs to open, soften and release. Working on the muscles of the neck (scalenes and sternocleidomastoid), muscles of the occipital ridge and muscles of the upper chest (pectoral) and upper back (trapezius and rhomboids) will help the breathing process and improve posture to aid good breathing. One of the characteristics of Parkinson's is a drooping head, and neck problems can ensue. Yoga can help strengthen and stretch the related areas, encouraging good posture and thus boosting confidence.

■ Body scan, levels of being

I often use this as a starting point in a class. It engages attention and brings mindfulness. It is a useful way to make a 'before and after' comparison. A similar process can be used at the end of class so that differences can be noted.

Instruction

1. Come into a comfortable lying (or seated) position.

2. Let your breathing steady.

3. Be aware of how your body feels.

4. Begin at your feet and notice any sensations in your feet: are they comfortable, heavy, warm? Is there any pain, stiffness, tightness? Are they numb?

5. Bring your awareness up through your legs, through your knees and thighs, and be aware of any sensations.

6. Continue up through your body, with awareness of what is happening today, where there is comfort or discomfort. You may notice areas that feel in need of stretching or softening, and even areas that feel good.

7. Move up through your middle, chest and back, noting what you feel.

8. Through your arms, shoulders, head and neck, which parts feel alive and which feel as if they need attention?

9. Become aware of your whole body, just as it is right now.

10. Now be aware of your energy level. Do you feel bright and alive, or tired and drained? Are you full of energy or depleted? You do not need to look for reasons why; this is just how you are now.

11. How are you feeling emotionally? Are you happy, angry, bored, feeling down, frustrated, calm? Again, do not look for reasons why, as this is a snapshot of how you are now.

12. Do you feel spiritually nurtured and connected with your higher self?

13. As you practise yoga, feel that your whole being can be brought into balance.

14. Move and stretch, ready to begin.

NECK RELEASE AND STRENGTHENING

These movements can be done either sitting or standing. It is good to do them at the beginning of class as a warm-up, but they can also be used as a 'wake-up' after relaxation.

First, attention must be paid to the position of the spine, encouraging an upright posture and lengthening up through the crown of the head. Encourage the shoulders to move downwards and to soften.

■ Rotations

Instruction

1. Turn the head along the central axis of the spine. Keeping in a level plane, moving first right and then left, coordinate the breathing with the movement.

2. Maintain a long spine, and rotate the neck only as far as can be comfortably reached – no straining.

3. Rotate the head to the right as if you are going to look over your shoulder.

4. Find the end of the range of movement and breathe into the stretch; visualise moving a tiny bit more.

5. Come back to the starting point with the spine upright and a feeling of a long neck.

6. Rotate to the left.

This rotation can also be done lying down, with the floor as a guide, and supported by a block or blanket that aligns the spine and keeps the neck long, to avoid over-arching.

Teaching focus

- Correct the line of the neck using gentle hand guidance, where needed.

- Observe whether there is any one-sidedness, but do not push the limited side; notice and wait.

- There should be no movement in the shoulders. Put your hands on the student's shoulders to steady if needed, or encourage with words.

- Visual imagery can help here. Ask the student to imagine that they can take their head all the way round like an owl, using their eyes as well.

- The chin should be kept level.

■ Side moves

Instruction

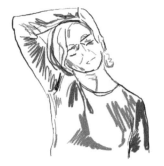

1. With an upright head, and neck and chin level, allow the head to move laterally, as if putting the right ear on the right shoulder. Avoid pressing down or straining, and let the neck travel within a pain-free range.

2. Return and repeat on the other side, noticing any differences or limitations, but do not try to correct and over-stretch.

Teaching focus

- There should be no movement in the shoulders or upper back. Put your hands on the student's shoulders to steady if needed, or encourage with words.

- If it is comfortable to do so, allow the student to stay in this position and breathe. Ask them to direct the breath into the stretch on the opposite side, to imagine the muscle lengthening, creating a space between the tip of the shoulder and the ear on the other side, and to then breathe into this space.

This whole exercise can be offered with an arm extended over and across the head so that a hand can be placed over the ear; in this way the movement has an added weight.

▦ Root of the neck

Instruction

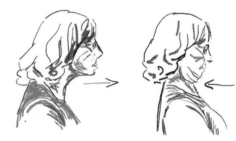

1. Push the chin forward, like a tortoise coming out of its shell.

2. Draw the head back, creating a double chin.

3. Repeat forwards and backwards.

This move mobilises the vertebrae and works the capitis muscles.

▦ Occipital ridge

Instruction

1. Begin by folding the arms to anchor the shoulders down.

2. Draw tiny circles with the tip of your nose and gradually spiral outwards so the movement increases.

3. Spiral back in again.

Teaching focus

- This should not result in throwing the head back or forward; the movement should be kept subtle.

EASING OUT THE SHOULDERS

▦ Simple shoulder rolls

These are a good starting point as shoulders are often rigid and tight.

Parkinson's note: Directing the students to simply shrug the shoulders around in a circle often results in them only moving their arms rather than their shoulders. This is where it is helpful to demonstrate clearly what you want the class to do, and do it with them. Walk around, and stand in front so that they can easily copy you. Sometimes you will find that people need you to show them by hands-on guiding, moving the shoulders gently in a circling action. The finger tips to shoulders version with elbow circling is easier to handle.

■ Lift and drop

This offers a good opportunity for release, using breath to facilitate the 'let go'.

Instruction

1. Lift the shoulders up around the ears with an in-breath.

2. Drop down with a sigh.

■ Hugs

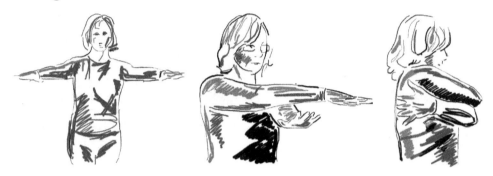

Instruction

1. Start with arms outstretched and then cross them over, bringing them in, to hold the opposite shoulder.

2. Creep your hands around and feel for your shoulder blades, giving yourself a big hug. This stretches the teres major, minor and infraspinatus. Note which arm is on top.

3. Take the arms out wide again and repeat, bringing the other arm on top.

■ Joint Freeing Pose (Pawanmuktasana)

All of the familiar Pawanmuktasana can be offered, and are particularly helpful in keeping the joints in action. They do often pose a problem with coordination, as the student may move joints other than those directed, which is due to faulty 'messaging'. Guide with demonstration and light-touch hands-on to show how the joint should move.

■ Arm twists

Instruction

1. With arms outstretched at shoulder height, release the shoulders downwards, with palms facing down.

2. On an in-breath rotate them, to palms facing up. Move between one position and the other with coordinated breathing, exhaling as the palms turn down.

Teaching focus

- Some students find it hard to maintain this position for more than one or two breaths, so allow rest time when needed.

▪ Swimming

Instruction

1. Breathe in, with hands together and elbows bent.

2. Push both arms forward on breathing out, as if swimming breaststroke.

3. Turn the palms up and open the arms wide, as you breathe in.

4. Repeat four times.

These are good general warm-ups in any class, and are essential before working more specifically into the shoulder and upper back area. See the postures in the shoulder and upper back section on page 97.

Further shoulder mobility and strength is gained in other classical postures, where movement and alignment work with the function of the whole body.

HANDS AND FINGERS

It is worth spending a little more time than usual to check out how each individual can manage wrist rotation, hand and finger exercises, as these areas are particularly affected by spasm, and where motor control is lost.

▪ Spread and clench

Instruction

1. Separate and spread the fingers wide; feel the stretch across the palm and between the fingers.

2. Make tight, tight fists or 'claws'.

3. Flick the fingers away sharply.

4. Repeat a few times for each hand.

▪ Shake

Loosely shake the hands as if you are shaking water off. This is good to do on a cold morning, to get the hands a little warmer.

Parkinson's note: Some students with Parkinson's have real problems with this and cannot loosen up enough to do the flicking. The same will apply if you offer foot loosening. Keep going and allow them to explore it anyway, and with practice, a little letting go can be achieved.

■ Up and down

Instruction

1. Start with the arms stretched forwards and palms facing down.

2. Push the heel of the hand away, and turn the fingers up towards the ceiling.

3. Flip them downwards. Up and down.

This can be varied using slow or fast movements, and a number of repeats. It can also be coordinated with the breathing – for example, two repeats for the inhale breath and two for the exhale.

Other variations are:

- Polishing: With the arms outstretched and palms facing down, move laterally from the wrist, out and in, as if they are moving on a flat surface.

- Wrist circling: With the hands in fists and the fists joined together, circle the wrists several times in both directions. Progress to doing this with the hands apart, but still circling the fists in the same direction.

Parkinson's note: The same challenge with coordination will occur here as with other joint-mobilising practices. In Parkinson's there is commonly difficulty with nerve transmission. You may observe that the student is moving the whole arm rather than just the wrist. Take time to work with this. Gently hold the arms still and encourage the work to happen in the wrists. Or give verbal direction, to bring this into focus and to isolate the wrist movement. This way we encourage full use of the body and retrain the nerve impulses.

■ Steeple

Instruction

1. Join the fingertips together.

2. Press them inwards and encourage the fingers to move towards each other, keeping the palms apart.

3. Encourage a stretch up into the length of the fingers and the finger joints.

4. Release the stretch, make the hands soft and repeat a few times.

Encourage the group to stop and release their hands whenever they feel the need.

Parkinson's/MS note: Prolonged practice can be tiring even for these hand/finger exercises; encourage awareness of any tension that might build up in the shoulders.

FEET

The feet are often affected by muscle spasm, joint stiffness, rigidity and poor circulation. Working on the feet is important for better standing and walking.

- Start by standing with good alignment, parallel feet, hips and knees. Have a chair nearby if needed for support. Explore your own feet with a range of practices such as:

- Awareness enquiry: Where is your weight? Left/right, toe/heel, inside edge/ outside edge?

- Inking: This brings aliveness and wakes up the nerve endings.

■ Inking

Instruction

1. Place one foot forward in a very deliberate step.

2. Feel the heel; roll your foot around along the outside edge and then onto the ball of the foot and through each toe. Imagine you are putting your foot on an ink pad and you have to get as much ink onto the sole of the foot as possible.

3. Press firmly through every part, and then do the same on the other foot.

4. Wriggle your toes. Lift them all up off the floor, if you can. Place the little toes down first, then all the others. (Not many people can actually do this, but it can be fun.)

Teaching focus

• Bring attention to the sense of aliveness experienced in the feet as the nerve endings are stimulated.

• Encourage the students to feel into both feet, and explore any differences they notice, any tingling, warmth, numbness, stiffness or immobility.

• This improves circulation.

■ High heel press

Instruction

1. Lift one heel and press the ball of the foot into the floor, then swap over to the other foot.

2. Move on to lift one foot as the other lowers. This also gets the knees moving a little, and is good for warming up if the feet are cold.

3. Awareness of the foot positions should be brought into all standing postures.

■ Make your feet talk

Basic stretches and joint rotation are essential. The wide range of commonly known Pawanmuktasana for the feet is useful. These can be done from a standing position to encourage strength and balance, or from a chair or floor seated position.

Contraindications of applied Ahimsa: Although these joint freeing moves are generally safe for everyone, they would be contraindicated if toe joints were swollen and painful, as they might be in rheumatoid arthritis, bunion or similar joint problems or plantar fasciitis. I would always recommend working within a pain-free range.

◼ Point and flex

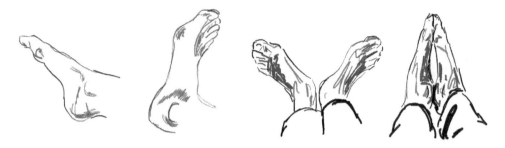

Instruction

1. Simply point the toes away, lengthening through the ankle, and then pull the toes up, as you push the heel away.

Teaching focus

- Bring attention to the movements felt in the lower leg, as this action involves far more than just the foot itself.

- Isolate the toe joint action by keeping the ankle down but the toes up, as in 'ankles down, toes down, toes up, ankles up'.

- Using a resistance band can really help strengthen the feet and toes, which is especially helpful for those who have difficulty in feeling what is happening. The student should place the band around the toes and ball of the foot and hold the ends firmly. They should action the movements by pushing and spreading the toes into and against the band. People with Parkinson's find this resistance helpful, but be careful of catapult action of suddenly released bands!

◼ Circling

Instruction

1. With both feet together, draw circles with your toes and ankles.

2. Try it with the feet apart and then move them both in the same direction (this is counterintuitive, but good for coordination and the brain).

◼ Flippers

Instruction

1. With the heels together, flex the ankles and pull the feet apart.

2. Draw the soles of the feet together. Try to join the little toes.

Teaching focus

- This tones and strengthens the flexor muscles in the sole of the foot, helping to combat flat feet. Again it is useful to draw attention to the action in the lower leg.

◾ Spread and scrunch

Instruction

1. Open out the toe joints as much as possible, and try to make a space between each toe.

2. Scrunch the toes up, as if making a 'fist' with your feet.

Teaching focus

- Although it is helpful in the first instance to sit with the group and to demonstrate, hands-on help may be needed. Physically moving the feet (check out permission first) can help the student to be more able to then do the movement alone.

- If there is little movement, add in visualising so that creative thinking can enhance the experience.

- Use humour to engage a light-hearted positive energy.

Parkinson's note: There is often a malfunction in motor control that limits activating a particular joint, and this may result in movement transferred to the joint above or below, as the student tries to follow the instruction only to find the message has been scrambled, so their knees and hips move instead of their ankles. This is where hands-on help and instruction to focus can really assist. Moving near to or in front of the student and doing the move so that they can follow is supportive. It can help to stabilise one joint – that is, the shoulder to enable the wrist to move, or to hold the hip or knee steady so that the foot can move.

SITTING WARM-UPS

As transferring from the floor to chair to standing can be a problem for some students, it is helpful to vary the programme so that some weeks there are fewer ups and downs.

I discovered 'Undulating' on a visit to America, and find that this simple spinal work can be fun and helps release tensions before class. Anita Boser (2007) invented this work, and it is suitable for anyone with limited movements as it encourages an exploration of movement and limitations.

Here is a simplified preliminary version. It can be done sitting on the floor, on a block in any comfortable cross-legged position, or with the legs bent and hands resting on the knees, or seated on a chair.

1. Sit upright on the 'sit' bones, the ischia.

2. Begin exhaling with a hollowing of the abdomen, rounding the back and drawing the abdominal muscles in.

3. Begin to arch the back, opening the chest, and breathe in.

4. Let the movement flow from one action to the opposite, hollowing and then rounding, extending and flexing.

5. Feel into the movement and notice any areas that are not moving or that feel stuck.

6. Focus on letting the movement begin from the stuck place and keep the spine moving into a 'C' shape, back and forth.

The next step would be to move from the 'C' shape into an 'S' shape. This is meant to be a free-form flowing movement; allow the group to play with it.

This can then be changed into a side-to-side 'C' shape action. Again, allow the students to explore the restrictions and keep the movements flowing.

The whole spine is energised during this process; the joints, muscles and fascia get a workout. As everyone is working within their own parameters, there are few contraindications to this flowing warm-up. It also encourages people to 'put their mind into their body' and to envisage the action as well as to physically feel it.

■ Side stretches

Sitting side stretches are a good way of connecting through the 'sit' bones, whether on a block on the floor or on a chair.

Instruction

1. Through the side bend the 'sit' bones should remain in contact with the floor, thus placing the stretch into the latissimus dorsi, obliques and intercostals.

2. From this position open up the ribcage and encourage breathing through the stretch.

3. Hold the arms downwards, finger tips on the floor to stabilise. Progress the stretch by extending an arm up and over the head.

Teaching focus

- Keep the 'sit' bones on the floor/block/chair.

- Root the tailbone into the ground, grow the spine long.

- Open up the side stretch and breathe into it.

- Grounding – keep the student's awareness down in their feet and conscious of their relationship with the ground.

■ Cat Pose (Marjariasana) warm-ups (known as Cat/Cow in the US)

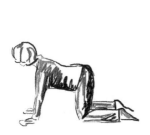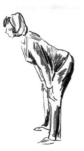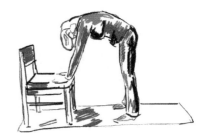

Cat Pose takes a little preparation as there may be varying problems and restrictions. Props need to be on hand. Offer rolled blankets for supporting inflexible ankles, folded mats or folded blankets to cushion knees, wedge-shaped blocks or folded blankets for wrists, particularly if there is carpel tunnel or arthritis. It sometimes takes time for students with Parkinson's to move onto the floor. In severely affected students, assistance may be needed in transitioning to the floor.

Instruction

1. On hands and knees, align the knees under the hips and wrists under the shoulders, inner elbows facing each other. Check that you have the correct spacing to enable the spine to flex and extend freely.

2. Bring awareness into the spine and tilt the pelvis downwards, lifting the tailbone on the inhale breath. Allow the upper spine to extend.

3. Move awareness into the pelvic floor, connect and contract slowly as you begin the pelvic curl, drawing the tailbone under, as you exhale.

Teaching focus

• This is the movement that all yoga teachers will recognise as an easy relaxing warm-up for the spine. As the group continue to work this posture, there is an opportunity to observe each individual and to work with them on the posture.

• Give permission to release the wrists any time they need to, and to come out of the pose when a rest is needed.

• Be sensitive to the fact that the group may not be able to sustain a kneeling position for too long.

Parkinson's note: In this pose coordination difficulties surface. You may see bent elbows, and rocking backwards and forwards from the hips instead of the spinal movement that we are expecting. This is where individual attention is important. Move alongside the student and state exactly what needs to happen – that is, 'Keep your hips over your knees and move your waist up and down'. Place a hand where you want the movement to be. Note when the movement changes and give encouragement; give a simple direction such as 'be still here' or 'lift here'. Encourage steadiness throughout the whole movement. Look for balance difficulties; core strength is also essential.

Contraindications are for knee problems, if there is pain or swelling, and similarly for wrists. You may find that this same action is still a problem a week later, so simply go over the same ground. This is due in part to a lack of dopamine.

CAT POSE PROGRESSIONS

From Cat Pose you can offer stretches and other poses. Cat Pose is useful to work some other strengthening asanas and warm-ups. Leg extensions from Cat Pose are useful for strengthening the lower back, legs and buttocks, and offer time to practise balancing.

■ Extend and curl

Stabilising on three points, without collapsing or dropping one hip, is the challenge. In order to do it, there has to be core strength. So, in preparation, engage the abdominal and pelvic floor muscles.

Instruction

1. Lift and extend one leg by sliding the toe along the floor to keep steady, and then lift and stretch. Lengthen the leg and push the heel away. Stay steady throughout the move, and try to keep the hips level.

2. Keep everything as stable as possible on the return journey.

3. Draw the leg right through and curl the spine. The nose towards the knee gives a natural balance to the action.

4. Repeat using the other leg.

This movement can also be done in the chair version (see page 200).

■ Arm strengthening

Instruction

1. With the hands and knees placed in the correct alignment, transfer the weight of the body forward, so the hands, arms and shoulders bear more weight. This enables you to get used to taking the weight onto the hands, and will help when transferring from lying to sitting to standing.

2. Rock the weight back into the knees, and then repeat the action a few more times.

■ Circles

Instruction

1. Rock forwards and then move the whole spine in a flat circle to the left.

2. Shift back and move up through the right, as if drawing a horizontal circle with your navel.

3. Then go the other way.

◼ Mini balance

Instruction

1. From Cat Pose, lift the right hand a few centimetres off the floor along with the opposite knee, so that there is balance on a diagonal basis.

Teaching focus

- Encourage the students to hold the balance. This challenges balance, strength and core strength.

◼ Side bends

Instruction

1. Walk your hands around to the right and then to the left, as if you are looking at your 'tail'.
2. Stretch along the sides of the body and open up the ribs.
3. Hold and breathe into the stretch.
4. Repeat a few times.

◼ Knee circles

Instruction

1. Stabilise over three points and lift one bent knee out to the side.
2. Lift the knee up out and around, moving the hip joint.
3. Repeat on the other leg.

CAT POSE ADAPTATIONS

These can be used if the student is unable to kneel.

Instruction

1. Using a chair, stand facing the chair and bend to rest the hands on the chair (blocks can be used to adjust height). Legs should be parallel. The spinal movement can be done from this position, but the legs may need to be slightly bent, if the hamstrings are tight. If the chair option is not suitable, a standing Cat Pose could be an alternative – that is, with knees slightly bent, bend forward a little to rest the hands on the thighs, just above the knees.
2. From this position start the spinal 'cat' movements.

Cat Pose is a wonderfully useful posture as it can be done by almost everyone and has the benefit of working the spine, easing back pain and improving coordination.

■ Hip sway in Cat Pose

Instruction

1. With the knees together and arms apart, swing the hips over towards the floor to the right, and then to the left. This creates a 'slalom'-type action, and is helpful in the ability to transfer to and from the floor.

LYING WARM-UPS

Starting the session in a lying-down position is always a popular option. It gives the student time to arrive, to put the journey aside and to steady the breathing. It allows the teacher time to observe the group and to judge their state of being. During this time students can be guided in bringing their energy into focus for the session. This is a good time to do 'body scan' awareness, and for the student to tune in and acknowledge what is happening for them physically, any aches and pains, tensions, trouble spots, their energy and emotional state. It is an opportunity for a snapshot of how things are now in the moment, and for them to feel that they can carry that awareness through into the whole practice.

■ Neck releases in a lying position

Alignment is still important even in the lying position, and the floor can offer a good guide for the spine, head and neck. Starting in semi-supine with the knees bent gives a comfortable way of working with the neck releasing, but brings different things into focus. The head needs to be supported until the neck is long and not over-arched, supported by one or more blocks if necessary. A head roll can be guided with awareness of the rotation on the axis of the spine, and having the head supported in this way can help with the release, as there is little effort in the action.

Contraindication: In elderly students there is often much rigidity in the neck – there may be arthritis or spondylitis, conditions that may be painful and restrictive, so it is important to work within a pain-free range and to allow the student to work within comfortable parameters, guiding gently to gain further movement. If the upper spine has kyphosis, it may be impossible to work this safely from a lying position, and sitting would be better.

Teaching focus

*   When working with limitations in the neck, it is helpful to use visualisation. Offer the idea that each rotation moves a little more, and that with each turn of the head there is a freeing of the cervical vertebrae; add visualisation, such as imagining the muscles are like elastic.

*   Ask the students to breathe into the stretch, to imagine it opening, softening and lengthening.

■ Hip releasing

A good place to start is the familiar Pawanmuktasana, circling the knees by guiding with the hands. There are many common variations and progressions to this releasing movement that a yoga teacher will be familiar with:

1. Circle the knees outwards and inwards, separately, and then together.

2. Keep one knee pulled in an out-breath, lifting the head to the knee, and repeat with each breath. Repeat on the other side.

3. With the knee pulled in, slide the other leg along the mat, and extend through the back of the leg, pushing the heel away.

4. Pull both knees in, curling into a ball to extend the spine.

All of this can be worked with breath coordination.

Parkinson's/MS note: It is sometimes helpful to assist with this, as there is often one-sided action. With permission, you can gently take the knee and move it in the correct way, until the student is ready to take over.

■ Rock the baby

This movement helps to work into the hips and sciatic area.

Instruction

1. In a sitting position either on the floor or on a chair, sit up tall.

2. Bring the right foot onto the left knee, and let the right knee fall out to the side, by allowing rotation in the hip. Do not force the knee into position.

3. Hold the knee in the right hand and the foot in the left, and lift the leg as far as is comfortable, as if you are cradling a baby. Be gentle.

4. Rock gently from side to side.

5. Repeat with the other leg.

More flexible people will be able to draw the leg up closer to the body.

WARM-UPS FOR COLD DAYS

Unless you have a beautifully heated room, there are sometimes cold winter days when being on the floor is just too cold. These days are when we practise standing dynamic warm-ups. These are good to get the circulation going and warm up hands and feet.

■ Swing arms

Instruction

1. Swing the arms, backwards and forwards, keeping the arms loose in the shoulder joints and moving freely. Coordinate with the breath – in with a forward and backward swing, and then out with another forward and backward swing.

Parkinson's/MS note: In Parkinson's the loss of arm swing is characteristic of the disease, but can be improved. Observe the group, to see where people cannot loosen or let go. Encourage that swingy puppet-arms feel. This can be worked into a forwards and backwards step. Step forwards as the arms swing up, and then shift the weight onto the back foot and let the arms naturally drop. Repeat with the other foot forward.

■ Swing twist

With a loose turn of the shoulders and upper body, allow the arms to hang loosely and to 'hit' the body where they land.

DYNAMIC BREATH WARM-UPS

These are done breathing in through the nose and out through the mouth.

Instruction

1. With an 'easy step' forward (see page 80), turn the shoulders and hips to the front.

2. Bring the arms up and hold the hands in fists in front of the chest, knuckles together, elbows lifted out to the sides.

3. Breathe in, and sharply pull the fists apart. Breathe out, snapping the fists back together.

4. Repeat five times. Bring the feet back together.

5. Step forward onto the other foot and repeat.

6. With the feet in the same position as before, arms straight out in front at shoulder height, on a sharp in-breath lift the arms up quickly, then bring them down on an exhale. Repeat five times.

7. Repeat with the other foot forward.

■ Facial exercises

Speech difficulties are a common problem in Parkinson's and MS, and a frozen facial expression can be a symptom of Parkinson's, so it is useful to at least keep the facial muscles active. This can be done in a lying position, to overcome any shyness. I usually put it in before relaxation, when people are mostly lying down.

Instruction

1. With your mouth, make an 'eee' shape; you don't need to make a sound, just pull your mouth into the shape. Let go and do it again five times.

2. Now try an 'ooo'. Repeat five times, releasing in between.

3. Now move between the 'eeee' and the 'ooo' shape. Repeat five times.

4. Clench your teeth together and release. Repeat five times.

5. Frown deeply and release. Repeat five times.

6. Arch your eyebrows up, as if you are surprised, and release. Repeat five times.

7. Move between a frown and surprise, and repeat five times.

8. Press your tongue to the roof of your mouth and release. Repeat five times.

9. Roll your tongue up, and release. Repeat five times.

■ Making sound

A mantra is great for encouraging good breathing and keeping the voice strong. Singing is encouraged for people with Parkinson's. Work with what is culturally appropriate in sound. Exploring the creation of sound through 'aum' means that you can introduce the sound without its devotional meaning.

I also explore sound using the vowel sounds, moving through 'aay', 'eee', 'iy', 'ohh', 'yoo', which takes away the need for it to sound beautiful. If the group are well bonded, you can have a lot of fun with making sounds. Use your imagination and simple song verses that would be well known to your group.

In planning any warm-ups, I usually consider movements that will awaken the spine, putting it through its paces and stimulating the nerve junctions. Flex, extend, rotate, lateral bends and swaying wake up the spine; add in joint freeing and overall stretching, and you are ready.

Posture and the spine

In Parkinson's there is a tendency for the posture to become increasingly flexed, known as the 'simian' posture. The head is held forwards, the spine becomes kyphosed, and the pelvis moves to posterior tilt, as flexion increases at the hips and knees. Trunk rotation and extension become more and more limited. Some muscles may gradually become contracted and shortened, and others lengthen but become ever more weak and unable to contract.

Poor posture contributes to breathing, speech and swallowing difficulties. Stiffness and rigidity make lying flat difficult, and sometimes a scoliosis develops. For MS students, working on the spine and improving inner strength will keep good posture and aid balance and improve joint mobility.

Yoga asana is an ideal form of movement to help maintain good posture. Core strength is vital, as is awareness of how one is standing and walking. Mountain Pose (Tadasana) is a good starting point to bring awareness of the standing posture. All of the asana practices should bring in an awareness of alignment, posture and positioning of the shoulders and head, but here are some postures to target the core muscles and flexibility of the spine.

Core strength and stability

The combination of abdominal muscles and pelvic floor make the inner core, and latissimus dorsi, gluteals, oblique abdominals and hip adductors make the outer core muscles. There is a great emphasis on building core strength, with the advent of the Pilates techniques that have shown how useful it is to keep these core muscles toned and working. Engaging the core muscles within yoga practice will increase the strength of the spine and improve the ability to get up and down out of a chair, for example. We can begin to bring awareness of these muscles in postures such as semi-supine and Cat Pose.

PELVIC FLOOR

The men in my groups often ask me if they have a pelvic floor! The answer is yes, of course, although it is structured differently. Personally, I always go into detail about the circles of muscle and how they need to be toned to function well, as this will help continence as well as being a key element in posture and strength.

For men this is the muscle group that lifts the testes, which sometimes needs an analogy. I describe it as like an aeroplane's undercarriage – imagine lifting the wheels up and tucking them in. I use a lot of hand gestures (to the amusement of my students, but they get the message).

For women it is easier to explain, as we use the same muscle group to stop the flow when urinating.

Imagine that you have two circles of muscle, one within the other. Draw in the inner ring up inside your body and then draw the outer ring up. Do this gently.

■ Mountain Pose (Tadasana) (standing well)

Good posture is essential for the health of the spine, nervous system, breathing and walking well. Posture has a bearing on the wear and tear of joints and helps us to avoid some of the related health complications.

Mountain Pose (Tadasana) is sometimes taught with the feet and toes together, but for a feeling of strength and balance, the parallel foot form is preferable.

Instruction

1. Stand with the feet parallel, so that they are in line under the knees, hips and shoulders.

2. Lengthen the spine. Imagine being drawn up from the crown of the head, and lengthen the tailbone down, like a dragon's tail. Don't tuck it under.

3. Let the shoulders soften and move them down and back.

Teaching focus

- Keep the alignment awareness active, in Mountain Pose or in any other standing pose. This means:

  - keeping in parallel alignment

  - keeping grounding through the feet and tailbone

  - paying attention to the position of the shoulders

  - paying attention to the position of head and neck – with the chin parallel to the floor

  - activating the core muscles

  - maintaining the length through the whole of the spine.

- Make time to give people individual attention, as they will all be different.

- Stand facing your student and mirror their posture. Tell them that you are going to do this, and then work together, balancing out the shoulders or any anomalies that you see, and get them to copy you. Give guidance with words at the same time, and use a light touch to adjust. For example, 'Drop this shoulder a little', 'Lengthen the back of your neck and tuck your chin in', 'Draw your ribs in'.

- When aligned and balanced as much as possible, direct the student to breathe along the spine up from the feet. Spread the breath into and around the ribcage.

- Mountain Pose (Tadasana) is a good starting point for many postures, but if standing is tiring or difficult for some, the same directions can be adapted for sitting.

■ Working the core in Mountain Pose (Tadasana)

Instruction

1. Stand in Mountain Pose (Tadasana), this time with the feet together.

2. Exhale and press the insides of the legs together.

3. Pull the pelvic floor up and in.

4. Press your hands in to the sides of your body.

5. Draw everything in and up, and hold.

■ Staff Pose (Dandasana) (sitting well)

With appropriate props in place, this posture offers an opportunity to build core strength.

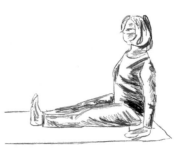

Instruction

1. Extend the heels and stretch through the hamstrings; gradually, it may be possible to take any under-the-knee support away.

2. Draw the trunk up tall; engage the pelvic floor and the abdominals.

3. Place the arms down on the floor firmly or with fingertips, or on supporting blocks or bricks. The whole body should be strong and taut.

4. Hold for a number of breaths (that can gradually be extended), then experience release and softness on letting go.

A version can also be offered from a chair with a couple of possibilities:

1. With knees bent and feet parallel, be aware of sitting up on the 'sit' bones. Hold the sides of the seat and raise one leg straight, lower it, and then try the other leg. This way we can notice whether we have one side more responsive or stronger than the other. Try both legs together.

2. Use two chairs facing each other and spaced so that straight legs can be supported. Raise the legs to the chair in front, as you would if you were on the floor (but take care that you are safe enough to sit this way).

Teaching focus

- Inner strength, core muscles active.

- Long spine.

- Feeling the strength of the ground and connecting to that, through the base of the spine.

- Move attention to, and root through, Muladhara.

- Breathe up through the spine, and grow tall.

- Offer 'hands-on' guidance for straightening the spine, placing your lower leg behind the student's spine to assist uprightness without pushing too much, so that they can feel what 'upright' is like.

- Offer hands-on assistance to ease the shoulders down, or to even up lopsidedness.

The posture can be progressed by extending the time it is held. You can add levels of difficulty with arm lifts. Lifting the arms in parallel while engaging the pelvic floor and abdominals will build strength and improve posture. Holding a block widthways and actively engaging the subscapularis and teres major, drawing the shoulders down, is another strength-building postural-improving move.

■ Inner core awareness in semi-supine

Instruction

1. Lying with the knees parallel and bent, place a supporting block under the head to keep good neck alignment.

2. As you exhale, pull the navel towards the spine, engaging the abdominal muscles, This will enable the back of the waist to press into the floor and the pelvis to tilt, as the pubic bone moves toward the head.

3. Release, and create a small natural arch under the waist on the inhale breath.

4. Practise this pelvic rocking action.

5. Actively use the abdominal muscles to initiate the movement, and tuck the tailbone under, and then release and feel as if you are rolling the tailbone out along the ground.

Teaching focus

- Offer this movement regularly so that students become accustomed to the feel of this muscle action.

■ Working the core in Cat Pose (or Cat/Cow Pose)

Instruction

1. Balance on all fours with the hands under the shoulders and knees under the hips. Check that the spacing is enough to let the spine move.

2. Begin to inhale and lift the tailbone, hollow the spine and lift the head.

3. On the exhale, draw the tailbone under, arch the back up and at the same time pull up the pelvic floor and draw the abdomen in.

4. Hold, and release on the inhale breath.

5. Repeat to become familiar with the action of the inner core.

MOVEMENTS OF THE SPINE

The spine can move in the following ways:

- Extension: back bending, maximal in lumbar, but also in cervical.

- Flexion: forward bending, maximal in cervical, but also in lumbar area.

- Rotation: twisting maximal in the upper thoracic.

- Lateral flexion: sideways bending, lumbar and cervical regions.

- Circumduction: swaying and circling.

To keep the spine mobile, we need to offer practices that cover the wide range of movements that the spine can make. By observation, we can assess where our students have rigidity or weakness. This does not necessarily need to be at the level of an osteopathic or medical examination. As a yoga teacher, you will 'see' where your class are struggling, and be able to plan a programme accordingly.

Instruction for some of these simple movements for mobilising the spine can be found on page 40 and pages 49–50.

Extension: back bends

Back bends are useful for keeping the spine strong and flexible, and for combating the 'simian' posture in Parkinson's. For MS students, they will be invaluable in maintaining strength in the spine. Standing and kneeling back bends have more possibility for bad technique. Gentle seated back bends offer a passive method of gaining flexibility and lying, where the floor provides good support for starting to build both flexibility and strength in postures such as Cobra and Locust.

■ Prone/face-down postures

This is a useful group of postures essential for strengthening the back and ensuring good shoulder positioning and strengthening for the upper thoracic. Encourage students to work within their own physical limits and within a pain-free range. Age, injury and kyphosis will all add limitations.

A folded blanket placed under the hips will offer comfort and support. Check whether the feet are able to lengthen and the top of the feet can rest on the floor. Offer a rolled blanket under the ankles for ease if this is not the case.

Be clear about the intention and goal of the posture – that is, to combat round shoulders, bring extension into the upper back, strengthen the muscles of the buttocks, lower back and core. The aim is *not* to lift up as high as possible, or to create as big a back bend as possible.

If you demonstrate the posture, do not show the best you can do – show what you expect your class to do.

■ Cobra Pose (Bhujangasana)

Cobra Pose is an amazingly strengthening posture that helps to maintain an upright strong spine; it aids in combating round-shoulderedness and stooping postures. Start with the simplest version so that people can gain confidence and feel that there is a level that they can achieve.

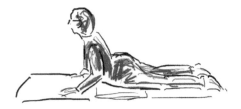 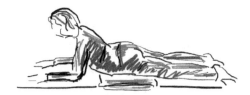

Instruction

Begin with Sphynx version:

1. Lie with the elbows placed under the shoulders and the forearms on the floor, providing a supported lift and curve to the upper back. In this position feel the active movement of the shoulder blades, down and back.

2. Keep the spine extending, so that the posture becomes active.

3. Follow with a release of the head that can hang forward to stretch the base of the neck.

4. Repeat this movement a few times. It can provide good loosening of the neck that is often held in tension.

For Cobra Pose:

1. Lie face down, bring your hands under your shoulders, draw the elbows back and the shoulder blades down your back; keep the legs parallel, feet pointing away.

2. Exhale, draw in the abdomen and engage the pelvic floor.

3. Let the nose travel forward and then lift the head away. Don't push the chin out, compressing the back of the neck; keep the back of the neck long.

4. Feel that the legs are strong, and use the buttocks and hamstrings to anchor you to the floor. With the shoulders pulling down and the shoulder blades feeling as if they are sliding down your back, explore how far the upper body can lift off the floor without using any pressure in your hands. This may not be very far.

5. Let the chest move back onto the floor and lower the head down, then the chin, nose, and then the forehead. Rest and practise abdominal breathing. Repeat to familiarise yourself with the effort needed and the technique.

To further the practice:

6. By using the breath to help the lift, begin to press into the hands to assist. Come up higher, but maintain the down shoulder position and upper back extension.

7. If lying on the floor is impossible, a more gentle back bend can be worked from the chair.

Teaching focus

- Pay attention to arm and shoulder strength, and where people may be struggling, encourage working within personal limits.

- Awareness in the upper back and hands/shoulder/elbow placement.

- Encourage by stating the benefits, such as 'feel strong and graceful'.

- Counteracts round shoulders and a humped spine.

- Activate the buttocks and legs.

- Encourage the lengthening and extending of the spine.

Parkinson's/MS note: Some may find that this is tough, as it requires strength and upper back mobility, so praise even the smallest changes. My experience is that this is often a posture where I see a lot of improvement over the weeks, and that improvement is built on in the standing postures. For those with MS, there may be overall weakness in the muscles that aid the push up. Allow the student to do whatever is possible, and give encouragement.

■ Chair back bend

Instruction

1. Sit tall towards the front of the chair, with feet and knees parallel.

2. Hold the back of the chair seat and anchor your tailbone down, as if you are growing it towards the floor.

3. Begin your back bend from the very base of the spine. Lift the spine up and the breastbone forward and arch the back.

4. Support the head and neck by tucking the chin in a little and lengthening the back of the neck. Keep the chest open and hold for four breaths.

5. Come out of the posture and release the head and neck forward.

Teaching focus

- Keep the breastbone lifted.

- Make allowances for kyphosis.

- Encourage the bend through the whole of the spine.

- Enjoy the release following the posture.

- Anahata chakra – heart-centred energy focus.

■ Standing back bend

This is contraindicated for some back problems, such as a strongly kyphosed spine and scoliosis. Work with it sensitively and steadily.

Instruction

1. Bend your knees, support your hips in the lower back, and keep the pelvis forward.

2. Lift the spine and keep the breastbone forward; keep the neck supported. Go only as far as feels safe and comfortable.

For the chair-supported version, experiment with a standing back bend similar to a Cobra stretch:

1. Stand behind the chair about 2 feet away, and hold the back.

2. Engage the core, lift and lengthen the spine and arch the back from the hips.

3. Lift the breastbone, and keep the chin slightly in, with the head supported.

■ Locust Pose (Shalabhasana) (leg lifts)

Instruction

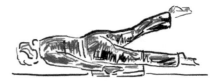

1. Place a blanket or pillow under the front of the body, if needed. Check that the tops of the feet are on the floor and long, and support with a rolled towel if needed.

2. Lie face down. Place your forehead down on the mat, arms down by your sides. Alternatively, place your elbows out and forward, to rest your head on your hands.

3. Exhale and draw the abdominal muscles in, toning the buttocks and back of the legs.

4. Without tipping over to the side, lift one leg, keeping it as strong and straight as possible. Lower it in a controlled way.

5. Repeat four times.

6. Do the same on the other leg.

Teaching focus

- Keep the whole body stable.

- The height of the leg lift doesn't matter as much as the feeling of strength extension.

- Check that there is no tipping over or outward turn of the leg. Make individual adjustment where needed.

- Swadisthana chakra, and lower back awareness.

- Feel into the front of the hip joint and imagine the leg lengthening away from that place.

If you are working individually, you can offer some hands-on correction for alignment and to discourage tilting to one side – for example, a hand placed on the lifted hip or gently holding the leg in place, while asking the student to connect to the muscles needed to do the job.

Progress to the full posture with both legs lifted, supported by a fist under the hip joint to provide leverage. Although this requires strength, the preparatory work will be of benefit even if no lift is achieved.

This is contraindicated for inguinal hernia and severe kyphosis.

■ Standing Locust Pose

If working on the floor is impossible, a wall- or chair-supported version can be offered.

Instruction

Using the wall:

1. Stand close to the wall and place your hands on the wall at shoulder height.
2. Keeping the pelvis facing the wall, lift one leg away at the back.
3. Hold it for a moment and bring it back in. Repeat four times.
4. Repeat with the other leg.

With chair support:

1. With the chair back facing you, hold the chair.
2. Keep the hips facing the back of the chair and lift one leg back and away.

Teaching focus

- Check that the body does not tip forward to give the feel of a leg lift.
- It doesn't matter how high or far the leg is lifted.
- Keep the core muscles engaged.
- Strength and stability.
- Swadhistana chakra.

Flexion: forward bending

Stretching and lengthening the muscles of the back of the body will provide a counter-pose to the back-bending asanas, but also help to work any rigid areas.

Contraindication: Forward folding is contraindicated for people with osteoporosis, high blood pressure, glaucoma or a detached retina.

■ Standing Forward Fold (Uttanasana)

The bending action for this posture will come from the hip joint, so that the spine can stay long throughout.

Instruction

1. First step. Stand in parallel, and feel where the hip joint is.

2. Offer a preliminary bend with the hand on the hip joint, and with knees bent.

3. Exhaling, bend from the hip joint in a hinging action. Fold over as far as is comfortable, and then come up to the start position, inhaling.

4. On an inhale breath, lift the arms up towards the ceiling, and lift and lengthen through the front of the body as well as the back.

5. Exhaling, bend from the hip joint, keeping the spine long and allowing the knees to bend.

6. Reach forward and then down. Let the hands and arms rest wherever is comfortable.

7. Come out on an in-breath and stretch the arms forward, and then bring the spine up.

8. Alternatively, from the folded position, come up by uncurling the spine.

9. Walk the hands up the legs to come out of the posture if the back needs support.

Teaching focus

- Keep the knees released unless the hamstrings are able to allow the legs to be straight.

- Check that the knees don't roll inwards.

- Be aware of the muscles that are used in completing this movement.

- Let each student work within their own limits.

- Don't hold for too long at first; work with going into the posture and coming out of it.

◼ Using the wall or a chair

This forward-bending action can be offered from seated position or using the wall or a chair (Paschimottanasana, Seated Forward Bend) for support.

◼ Wall- or chair-supported bend

Whether you use a wall or a chair depends on the height of the student. The wall is usually better for taller people.

Instruction

1. Stand about 1 metre away from the wall, and place your hands on the wall at shoulder height. Adjust the position of your feet to get the best alignment for the spine – they can be a little wider than your hips. Explore what is comfortable.

2. Keep your knees bent if the hamstrings are tight.

3. Walk the hands up or down the wall until there is a feeling of comfortable supported stretch.

Teaching focus

*   Allow each student to explore their own limits.

*   Explore the distance, by moving further away from the wall.

*   Let the student begin with bent knees if necessary, and work towards straightening them gradually.

*   Look for body sagging, and encourage work into the abdominals, and check the shoulder position.

*   Check that the heels are down – a wedge-shaped block might help if there is strong shortening of the Achilles tendon.

*   Bring attention to the feet.

MS note: For some people with MS, numbness is an issue. This affects balance and stability and therefore needs to be considered in the standing postures. Not being able to feel the feet will impact on how the other muscles are moved and used, so individual attention and adjustments to alignment are essential. Here you are playing the part of giving feedback that is lacking in the nervous system.

▪ Seated Forward Bend (Paschimottanasana), on a chair

Instruction

1. With the feet parallel and placed on blocks, if that helps the feet to feel grounded, lift the arms in parallel, lengthening the torso and spine.

2. Forward bend from the hips on the exhale breath. Move into the bend slowly, going all the way down, hands to feet, or as far as they will go.

3. To progress, this posture could be worked more slowly, stopping halfway with the spine and arms horizontal with the floor, inhaling and exhaling on bending further.

4. To come out of the posture, lift and extend the arms up and forwards first, creating a horizontal line with the arms and the spine.

5. Lift all the way up and then relax.

6. If this is too strenuous, lift the spine with the arms in a soft relaxed position.

▉ Seated Forward Bend (Paschimottanasana), on the floor

Props are helpful in this posture – a block to sit on to enable a better bend if the hip joints are tight, or a rolled blanket to support under the knees if the hamstrings are tight and the legs cannot be comfortably straight, or a strap to help facilitate alignment of the spine.

Instruction

1. Sit on the block. Feel for the 'sit' bones and connect into them.

2. Take note of the knees and whether they want to bend; support underneath them with the rolled blanket if necessary.

3. Place the strap around the soles of the feet and leave the ends loose beside the legs.

4. Sit up tall and breathe in.

5. Lift the arms up to lift up the ribs, and reach up.

6. Hinge at the hip and bend forwards.

7. Let the knees bend.

8. Imagine you are going to lie along your legs. Go as far as you can and hold the ends of the strap, or hold your legs.

9. Move a little further into the stretch.

10. Come out by lifting the arms up again and sitting upright, or let the arms drop and return to upright in a softer way.

This is contraindicated if there is osteoporosis, and hiatus hernia may also prove problematic if acute.

Teaching focus

• Go only as far as is comfortable.

• Imagine a long line down the front of the body, and keep the line long.

• Let the crown of the head move towards the feet, not the knees.

• Swadistana chakra.

• Breathe along the stretch, imagine light and space in the spine.

• Avoid poking the chin forward, and keep the back of the neck long.

Parkinson's note: Those with severe kyphosis should focus on extending the upper back and avoid 'crouching' over. Give guidance for the position of the head and neck.

■ Apanasana

This easy flexion posture is a great way to begin to warm up and to release tension in the lower back.

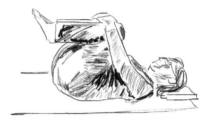

Instruction

1. Lie flat on the floor. Support the head with a block to keep a length in the neck. This pose can also be started in a semi-supine position.

2. Bend one knee, reach and clasp it in your hands, and fold it towards your body, as you exhale. Hug the knee and inhale, exhale again and lift your head up towards your knee.

3. Inhale and put your head back on the block, exhale and lift it towards the knee.

4. Repeat this action five times.

5. Slide the leg away, and draw the other leg in.

6. Repeat the movements and breathing.

7. Draw both knees up together and hug them in on the exhale breath. Hold and inhale.

8. Exhale and lift the head to both knees. Inhale and lower the head back to the floor.

Teaching focus

- Check for the head/neck position and support where needed.

- Observe any difference in mobility in right and left.

- Imagine breathing into the whole length of the spine.

- Imagine the muscles lengthening and stretching like elastic.

Rotation

Twisting postures enable the small joints of the spine to be mobilised. Yoga offers standing, sitting and lying versions of this same action. Each offer something a little different and are more passive or active depending on application.

▓ Standing twists

The important thing about this posture is to bring attention to the length and alignment of the spine and to discourage forward or back bending that is often seen as people try to attain a full twist. This move can be offered in several ways.

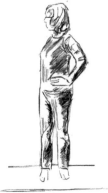

Instruction

Beginning with hands on hips, and spine upright, this is an exploration rather than a posture offered with attention to correct alignment:

1. Allow the whole body to twist from the feet and ankles upwards. This way you can experience the twisting, noticing whether there is an unpleasant pressure in the knees or any other places. This is not a very effective twist and can easily be detrimental, so we are using it here for a comparison. We can see how much of the twist is actually in the hips and legs rather than in the spine.

The next step would be to bring in the 'rules' for good alignment in standing twist:

2. Keep a long upright spine, keeping its natural curve, but staying with the idea of an upright pole.

3. Keep the hips facing front (imagine that your hip bones are like car headlights).

4. Let the spine turn, feeling this mostly in the upper body, as the hips stay facing forward.

5. Notice the limitation, don't push or strain, but rather use the inhale breath to grow taller and the exhale breath to turn a little more. The teacher will encourage this with guiding words, reminding you not to force the pose.

6. Repeat this two or three times, on each side.

Teaching focus

- Remind the class of the benefits of this movement: mobilising the spine is essential for good posture, movement and balance; twisting stimulates blood flow and stimulates nerve function.

◼ Twisting posture, chair version

This twisting posture can also be offered in seated form, which is useful for those who cannot stand for an extended time are unable to balance well enough, or if there is incidence of low blood pressure. It helps to stabilise the hips.

Instruction

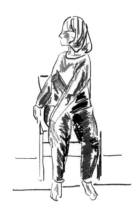

1. Using a chair, let the student sit towards the front to give room for the turn.

2. Sit up on the ischia (or 'sit' bones) to enable an upright posture rather than a slumped back position.

3. Turn, coordinating the breath with the movement as described above, taking the arm across the body right hand to left knee; the left hand can move around towards the back of the chair. Keeping the spine upright, encourage the tailbone to lengthen and the crown of the head grow towards the ceiling.

Some alternatives:

1. An option that gives more stretch is to sit sideways on the chair so that the back of the chair is to the side of the body. Turn toward the back of the chair and hold it, using it to aid the turn.

2. Using a block in both the standing or sitting twist aids the upper back and shoulder positioning – hold a firm block widthways out at shoulder height, draw the shoulders down and press the base of the little finger into the block (supination).

3. With the spine long and working with breath coordination, let the turn begin from the thoracic spine. This helps to keep the spacing and brings strength and steadiness.

Teaching focus

- In both standing and sitting versions it is helpful for a little hands-on support. Hands on shoulders encourages the student to open, and this should be a very light touch, as once the direction is given with the hands, the student will often very readily respond, and can manage further movement.

- Hands-on guidance can be helpful when there is a tendency for round shoulders or pulling away from the upright stance we want to encourage.

- Breathing up the spine in a spiral action – feel that this is bringing prana into the spinal column.

- Lengthening both at the tail and crown – imagine creating spaces between the vertebrae.

- Good positioning of the shoulders to aid pectoral stretch and to act as an antidote to round shoulders.

■ Half Spinal Twist Pose (Ardha Matsyendrasana) (seated twist)

This is a modification of the full practice familiar to all yoga teachers. Here we will explore easy stages, so that there is something that every individual can achieve, however immobile they may be. This asana offers further opportunities to work the spine and to improve posture, as well as improving the mobility of the spine, working the facet joints and energising the whole structure. All of the twisting postures, whether seated or lying, act on the digestive organs by pressure and massage action throughout the abdomen. This improves peristalsis, enabling more efficient movement of food though the system (in yoga terms, improved Apana flow and therefore elimination). Manipura chakra is stimulated and energised.

Instruction

1. From the supported seating position on the floor, use blocks under the 'sit' bones and a block or blanket under the knees, as described in Staff Pose (Dandasana) (see page 60).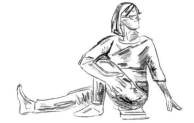

2. With the spine upright, turn the torso to each side alternately.

3. Place both hands on the floor to the side.

4. Do this slowly in your own time. This will give the teacher time to observe and offer support for each individual. Breathe with the movement, turning on the out-breath.

5. Draw up the right knee, place the foot next to the left knee, hold on to the knee with both hands and draw the spine up and sit up.

6. Hold the knee with the left hand and extend the right hand forward at shoulder height.

7. Turn towards the knee, drawing it as close to the body as possible, as you sweep the right arm around to the back, placing that hand on the ground or on a block or perched on fingertips.

8. Let the head and neck join in the movement to look back over the shoulder.

9. Use the eye muscles as well. Hold and breathe in, encourage a little more turn on the out-breath, return and repeat with the left knee bent and right leg straight.

10. Cross the foot over the knee and repeat the twist with the same instruction, focus and guidance.

Some students may attempt the full posture but it may require more hands-on help and care with the spinal posture. Note that the leg position of the full posture may be contraindicated for some types of hip replacement. Remember that the object of practice is not achievement of the full posture, but practise enough to bring health benefits.

Teaching focus

- The spine should remain upright, and not slump back, even if this means a less strong turn.

- Encourage releasing and turning on the out-breath.

- Breathing up and down the spine, visualise the twisting action as an energy flowing up and down.

- Stay anchored in the tailbone and 'sit' bones.

- Encourage the placement of the abdomen against the leg, feeling the breath in the belly creating a massage action.

- Energising Manipura chakra.

■ Lying twists

Among movements essential for mobilising the spine are twisting postures. These moves not only move facet joints of the spine, but also work in a wringing massage action on the intestinal tract. This stimulates samana vayu and apana vayu, helps peristalsis and can help relieve constipation that is commonly found in both Parkinson's and MS. These movements help in combating the rigidity in spinal muscles common in Parkinson's.

Instruction offered in stages

1. From a semi-supine position, with arms either outstretched along the floor or cupped behind the head, and with the knees together, ease the knees over to the left, just a little way at first; return and move to the right.

2. Repeat a few times so that the action becomes familiar.

3. Then take the knees as far over to the floor as is possible, keeping both shoulders down. Let the movements happen within a comfortable range.

4. Going further, bend the right knee in and straighten the left leg.

5. Stretch the right arm along the floor.

6. Put the left hand on the right knee.

7. Guide the right knee over to the left, and allow the bent knee to go over as far as is possible.

8. For holding in this position, you could be supported with blocks under the knee in the end position, to give time for releasing into the posture.

Teaching focus

- Check correct alignment, and offer support for the head and knee.

- Breathe into the space between the hip and armpit, and visualise lengthening.

- Allow the hip to release downwards.

- Keep the shoulders on the floor.

Parkinson's/MS note: This posture may take a little time to prepare, but it is worth the effort. Almost everyone can gain some progress and actually enjoy the stretch. If a student cannot get down to the floor, a similar twist can be accessed sitting with the legs to the side, on a chair. Both arms begin palms together, stretched forward at shoulder height (or hands on hips), and then turning the upper body and opening the arms out. The teacher can assist by checking that the spine is upright, and encouraging turning from the breastbone.

Lateral flexion: side bending

The side stretch lengthens through the latissimus dorsi and opens up the intercostal muscles as well as providing a side-bend action for the spine. This is a simple version that can be offered free-standing or that can be done from a chair.

Instruction

1. Stand with the back of a chair facing you (for support if needed), with your feet apart and arms down by the sides.

2. Bend to the side, by sliding one hand down the leg, just as far as you can go, keeping the spine as if you are standing with your back against the wall.

3. If there is wall space in the room, try practising against the wall. This will provide extra support, and by keeping the hips and shoulders against the wall, this focuses movement in the spine.

4. The posture can then be extended by lifting one arm on the inhale breath and bending to the side, to follow through.

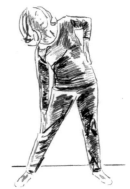

5. Use repeated movements in the first instance, and then add holding for a number of breaths – three or four is often enough to build stability. Early release if needed.

6. If sitting, check that the spine is upright to begin with. Hold the side of the seat and bend to that side. The arm can be raised to extend the stretch.

More side bending asana are described in the 'Superstretches' section (see pages 151–176) for Gate Pose and Triangle Pose.

It is likely that both Parkinson's and MS students will need support and feedback, as with rigidity and spasm, faulty messaging and numbness, it is often the case that students are not clear of their body position. Give encouragement and hands-on guidance.

Circumduction

Swaying is integrated into a few yoga movements. Within the Pawanmuktasana series we have the body roll and Tiryaka Kati Chakrasana (Waist Rotating Pose). These involve complex muscle movements and as such have great value in mobility. They are contraindicated for anyone with a history of disc problems, prolapsed discs or degenerative conditions of the spine. The twisting and bending action is the most challenging and complex action of the spine, and so caution is required if there is history of injury.

▇ Body roll

Begin with gentle mild versions to explore what is possible, starting with small circles at first.

Instruction

1. Stand or sit. Place your hands on your waist; the knees can be slightly bent.

2. Breathe in, and on an exhale turn to the right, lean forward and roll your body around to the front, and then begin to inhale as you lift up to the left.

3. Continue the rolling movement, coordinating with your breathing. Do this four times.

4. Stop, and then repeat the whole thing, going in the other direction.

Try to make the movement as smooth as you can.

▇ Stir the pot

Instruction

1. Stand or sit with your feet apart, knees slightly bent.

2. With your elbows bent, clasp your hands and breathe in.

3. Turn to the right and reach your arms forward, as if you are stirring a large pot.

4. Move the arms out in a wide flat circle to the front, and then pull them back in as you return.

5. Go round again. Repeat four times.

6. Circle in the other direction.

Teaching focus

• Check for any back problems.

• Work in a pain-free range.

• This posture has a warming effect as it massages around the solar plexus area.

• Focus on the Manipura chakra, fire centre.

Parkinson's/MS note: Keep a close eye on possible balance issues.

The movements described in this section help to keep the spine fully mobile. The most useful ones are the back-bending extension actions with work and awareness of core strength.

From a subtle energy point of view, it is thought that when we bend and flex the spine, we begin to awaken and enliven the chakra centres, and the life force within them, in preparation for more focused meditation work. A more mundane viewpoint might be that we are stimulating the nerve plexuses, and bringing blood flow to those parts of the spine. Whatever your viewpoint, we bring life, energy, strength and vitality to the body and mind.

Strength and stability

Immobility in the hips and pelvic areas can severely limit walking. In both Parkinson's and MS there may be instability throughout the lower body, and so the standing postures will help with strengthening the legs. In almost all yoga practices, activating the core muscles is preferable and even helpful. It keeps the integrity of the posture and spine, enables the limbs to operate more powerfully, and may prevent back pain.

If we are weak in the hips and legs, we are generally disempowered. Phrases such as 'standing on your own two feet', 'stand up for yourself' and 'had the legs taken from under me' reflect the importance of having strength in the legs and the ability to walk and move. If we can walk and move, we can explore, interact with others and feel independent. Imagine what it is like if you can't run away, or you freeze when you want to move fast. This is the reality of many with Parkinson's and MS, and with it comes fear and an undermining of confidence. These are issues of the Muladhara chakra. For those who cannot stand for too long, sitting and supine postures can do similar work and connect into the Muladhara energy centre. Linking asana practice with encouraging affirmations consolidates the work.

Remember that one of the side effects of the rigidity of Parkinson's is low blood pressure, and so many find standing for even short lengths of time uncomfortable, and may even begin to feel unwell. Good guidelines to avoid this are:

- Always offer the option of taking the postures in the adapted sitting form.

- Place a chair within easy reach, even if the student's balance is good.

- Avoid offering a long sequence of standing postures without rest.

- Always give permission to stop and to sit when necessary.

Many people with MS have issues in standing without sticks or support, so many of he practices that follow will need to be worked from a chair, or another means of stretching the body in a similar way should be found. For example, stretching the hamstrings could be worked in a semi-supine position or from a chair.

STANDING AND STEPPING

One of the key issues for Parkinson's disease is that the gait changes greatly – this is one of the defining symptoms of the disease. Bringing confidence and awareness to this function will be of real benefit to anyone with Parkinson's. In general, the stride becomes shortened and a shuffling walk develops. This is usually accompanied by a drooped head position.

When offering a programme of yoga, alignment and posture are key to many of the standing asanas. Promoting confidence in stepping and standing can make noticeable differences in posture that in turn brings many health benefits. Simply standing well can ward off the wear and tear instigated by poor function of the joints that often results in arthritis, joint pain and mobility problems.

As we know, yoga is best done barefoot – it promotes awareness in the feet, allows the feet to be worked fully and is safer, especially in the standing postures. However, there are some instances where students may not want to have bare feet. These may be where they get cold and numb if barefoot, or where they have foot swelling and therefore difficulty in getting their shoes back on after class. In these cases I permit working in shoes, preferably soft flexible ones, or socks, while in class, but encourage them to work barefoot in home practice. This does mean that they lose out on valuable foot exercises, but it is their choice.

▓ Mountain Pose (Tadasana)

Good posture is essential for the health of the spine, nervous system, breathing and walking well. This, in turn, has a bearing on the wear and tear of joints, and helps us to avoid some of the health complications that illness in any of these areas would bring.

This is more important in both Parkinson's and MS than it is in a general class.

Keep the alignment, with your awareness active, in Mountain Pose or any other standing posture. This means:

- keeping the body in parallel alignment, aligning through the feet, knees, hips and shoulders

- keeping grounding through the feet and tailbone

- paying attention to the position of the shoulders, drawing them down and back to open the chest

- paying attention to the position of the head and neck, keeping the chin level and the neck long

- activating the core muscles

- maintaining length through the whole of the spine, while at the same time maintaining its natural curves.

From here, breathe along the spine up from the feet, spreading the breath into and around the ribcage.

Mountain Pose is a good starting point for many postures, but if standing is tiring or difficult for some, the same focus can be adapted for sitting.

▓ Swaying Palm

From Mountain Pose (Tadasana), we can encourage a stretch through the sides of the body.

Instruction

1. Lift the arms in parallel and reach upwards.

2. Lengthen through the left then the right as a warm-up.

3. Ease into bending gently to each side.

Teaching focus

- Focus the class into feeling their way into this, easing into the swaying movements, staying within their own comfortable parameters.

- Check for any limitation in shoulder extension, and keep the focus on the movement of the spine rather than on the lift of the arms. If there is shoulder injury, frozen shoulder or severe kyphosis, the movement may be limited.

- Check that there is no forcing through any joint that is limited in this way.

- If there is pain in any movement, encourage working within a pain-free range; offer a hands-on-hips version or arms down by the sides instead.

- Bear in mind that in an older population the spine may already be changing its shape and its curves, and make allowances for this.

Other variations:

- Use a block to keep the spacing – it adds another dimension to strengthening the arms if we add a direction to squeeze the block.

- Bring awareness of the pelvic floor to provide more strength, stability and grounding, and a sense of 'earthing' through the base chakra, and flow of Apana.

- Swaying Palm can be offered from a chair, taking care that the student is safe enough to side bend.

▨ Awareness in walking

I have included this exercise, as practice and awareness builds confidence and improves stability, although it is really a moving meditation.

It is useful to stand next to a wall and to use a hand for support, until full confidence is gained.

Instruction

1. First bring full attention into the feet, using the 'inking' exercise (see page 47).

2. Place the hands on the hips and step forwards in slow motion.

3. Notice where in your body you initiate this movement. Be aware of how you lift the back foot and carry it forwards.

4. Keep your attention on how this foot connects with the ground and how your weight is transferred.

5. Continue in this way, and then turn around, so that the wall is on the other side.

Parkinson's note: People with Parkinson's often find that they don't place the heel down first when walking. It is therefore important to draw attention to which part of the foot strikes the ground first, and how you transfer your weight from the back foot to the front foot. Spreading your weight around the outside edge of the front foot, feeling it connect to the floor and waiting until you feel steady before thinking of taking another step, offers an awareness that can carry into everyday walking.

◼ Walking on tiptoes/heels

This strengthens the feet and toes. Do this on a mat with a chair for support.

1. Rise up onto tiptoes and take a few steps forwards, in a 'stompy' way, pressing the ball of the foot into the floor on each step.

2. Try walking backwards.

3. Tread forwards on your heels. And then backwards.

Try it without the chair.

◼ The easy step

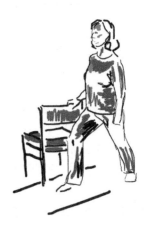

A chair can be used for support. In MS as well as Parkinson's, balance is often affected, so providing support builds confidence as well as strengthening the muscle groups and body-brain messaging. Make sure that the chair is not able to slip away if grabbed.

Instruction

1. Stand alongside the chair, the back of the chair nearest your hand.

2. Take a comfortable step forward (this enables the teacher to see what you can do easily). Most of the standing postures can be built from here.

3. If you gradually 'open out the step', this will promote a wider stance. It may be helpful to have some kind of measure, a stick, a belt or a line drawn on the mat. Try to move your foot position to that length if possible. If these tools are not available, step forward and then place a block on the ground 10 cm or so in front of your toes, and then step up to the block (the stride is achieved much more easily).

This will encourage and bring a sense of achievement and confidence, and can be used for the Warrior and Triangle Poses.

Parkinson's note: In many people with Parkinson's, body memory is an issue. Don't be afraid to go over the same ground each week.

Teaching focus

- From this position, bring the focus into the feel of the hamstring stretch, and encourage connection through the outside edge of the back foot into the ground.

- Give permission to hold the chair.

- Explore transferring the weight onto the forward foot, and then shift it back. This enables the student to develop proprioception and balancing skills.

- Gradually encourage the back foot to lift, promoting a small but safe balance.

- Work with this same posture over the weeks to build strength and confidence.

■ Warrior Pose 1 (Virabhadrasana I)

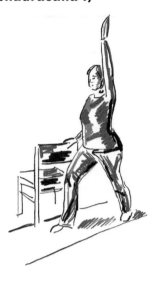

The Warrior group of postures are helpful in bringing stability and building strength, as they involve the ability to both ground and balance. They strengthen the legs, arms and shoulders, and promote confidence.

Instruction

1. In 'The easy step' position (see page 80), and with the back of a chair alongside that can easily be held for balance, look down and align your feet. Keep the feet parallel, hip-width apart, hips facing the front of the mat.

2. Practise bending the forward knee, checking that it doesn't travel beyond the ankle, and the knee moves towards the second toe, making a right angle at the knee, if this is achievable.

3. Engage the core muscles.

4. When aligned, hold the back of the chair with one hand, and lift the other arm. Both can be lifted when there is steadiness.

Teaching focus

*   Core muscle engagement.

*   Releases shoulder tension. Offer other arm positions – palms together in front of the chest, for example, or releasing the shoulders down and out so that there is more softness in the trapezius.

*   Stay connected to the floor – encourage sure-footedness, anchoring into the ground.

*   Check that the knee doesn't roll inwards.

*   With the chest open, practise full breathing.

*   Strength, stability, courage and balance.

■ Warrior Pose 1, variations

Instruction

1. Inhale and extend your arms upwards and in a long diagonal, lean forward – create one long line from the feet up through the straight leg, spine and arms.

2. Open the arms out at shoulder height (to help with balance).

■ Arm swings in Warrior Pose 1

In Parkinson's, people lose the ability to coordinate their shoulder movement with the pelvis, which is noticeable in walking where there is a limited natural arm swing. Encourage this action by using it in Warrior Pose 1.

Instruction

1. From Warrior Pose 1 leg position, keep the upper body facing the front.

2. Breathe in and stretch both arms forwards, to shoulder height.

3. Breathe out and take one arm back.

4. Using the breath to coordinate, let the arms change places, one back, one forward.

■ Warrior Pose 2 (Virabhadrasana II)

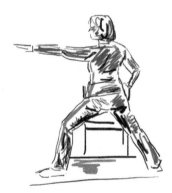

Instruction

1. Start with your feet in the same position as Warrior Pose 1, with the chair placed with the back in the centre of the long side of the mat. Turn the hips to square up with the back of the chair, and hold it with both hands.

2. Engage the pelvic floor and core muscles.

3. Bend the forward knee at a right angle.

4. Lift the forward arm to shoulder height, and if the posture is steady, let go of the chair and lift the other arm; if not, keep hold of the chair.

5. Turn your head and look back along the arm, checking that it is at shoulder height and not drooping.

6. Look forward along the front arm.

7. Return easily and gracefully, placing your hands back on the chair.

8. Adjust your foot position and repeat on the other side.

Ahimsa caution: Do not force the hips to open. Try to maintain the alignment of the forward foot and knee, and allow the student's own flexibility to guide where the hip position will be.

Teaching focus

- Long spine.
- Core muscles.
- Alignment.
- Grounding.
- Strong legs.
- Observe the relationship between the legs, back and shoulders.
- Keep the shoulders down and back, and soften.

▮ Warrior Pose 2, seated version

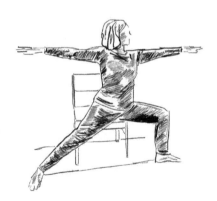

Instruction

For those unable to sustain balance in a standing position:

1. Sit on the front edge of the chair with the left leg bent and angled out to the side. The 'sit' bones should be near to the front of the chair. Check the stability of the chair – you may need to steady yourself using your arms.

2. Slide the right leg straight and plant the foot firmly on the floor, turning the ankle to do this.

3. Once the leg position is in place, engage the core muscles for strength.

4. Lift the arms up to shoulder height, palms facing down.

5. With the head upright and neck long, look along the line of the arm and hand to complete the posture.

■ Simple lunges

When standing postures are familiar, we can begin to introduce the idea that the feet can establish a solid stable base and that the body is able to move from that stable base.

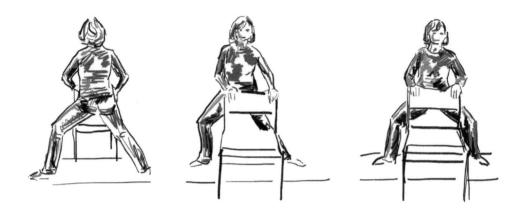

Instruction

1. Stand facing the back of the chair back, with hands on the chair back, feet apart and angled outwards, taking care to align the knees to track towards the foot.

2. Bend one knee in a gentle lunging action, let the knee travel as far as is comfortable, and then straighten the leg.

3. Do the action on the other side. This is a flowing move from one side to the other, bending and straightening alternately.

4. Progress the posture to bring the arms into a crescent moon shape by holding the chair with the left hand, bending the right knee and lifting the right arm to stretch over to the left, over the straight leg. Repeat on the other side.

5. Hold the chair with the left hand and bend the right knee.

6. Lift the right arm and stretch over to the left, over the straight leg.

7. Repeat on the other side.

Teaching focus

- It is useful for the teacher to show this first, and to do it with the group before giving any individual guidance. When the class is confident, add in breathing to coordinate and awareness of the pelvic floor.

- Encourage rhythmic movement, easing the knee and hip joints.

- Emphasise working within one's own limits and being pain-free.

■ Extended Side Angle Pose (Utthita Parsvakonasana) (bent-knee side stretch)

This posture is both strenuous and complex; it requires mental focus, some strength and stability in the hips and legs, but it is worth including for the challenge that it will bring.

Instruction

1. Place the chair on the mat so that it won't slip.

2. Take a wide stride (five foot lengths), and place one foot on the floor in front of the chair so that when the knee bends, it is against the seat of the chair.

3. Lunge the knee towards the seat and rest against it for steadiness. From here, work in stages towards the final posture.

4. Rest the elbow on the knee (or on the chair seat) and place the other hand on the ankle. Then practise rotating the body as the arm is lifted out and up, turning the chest and shoulders outwards.

5. Place the hand on the hip and continue to rotate the breastbone to align the shoulders.

6. Raise the arm in a straight line upwards, and eventually take it over the head, alongside the ear.

7. Come out of the posture in a steady way: bring the arm down and use the chair to push against to straighten the leg if needed.

Teaching focus

- Teachers should not at any point force or push a student, but give instruction by words and gentle hands-on guidance.
- Bring attention to the feet and ensure that they are stable.
- Give permission to stop at any time.
- Work within the student's comfortable range and encourage them to explore further.
- Breathe into the stretch.
- Open the chest and align the shoulders.
- Give lots of encouragement.
- Afterwards, rest in an easy forward fold.

■ Adapted Extended Side Angle Pose (Utthita Parvakonasana), using a chair

This is a physically complex posture. The challenge it provides is stimulating as the brain has to multi-task to achieve it, working the nerve pathways.

Instruction

1. Place the chair with the seat facing you.

2. Stand 60 cm (2 feet) or so away from the chair – this will give a stretch to the hamstrings.

3. Place the right foot up on the chair; for taller people, a block may be needed to adjust the height. Always check for stability of the chair.

4. Place your hands on either side of the foot, leaning the body down along the leg, but do not hunch over it – stay long in the spine.

5. Inhale and lift the left arm out to the side at shoulder height.

6. Exhale, then breathe in and turn the body – imagine leading by the breastbone and turn the body rather than move the arm. Let the head follow, if there is mobility.

7. Hold and breathe easily.

8. Repeat on the other side.

■ Revolved Side Angle Pose (Parivritta Parsvakonasana), reverse version

Instruction

1. Keep the left hand next to the right foot on the chair and lift the right arm, so that you are turning in towards the right knee.

Teaching focus

- These are complex postures, with or without a chair. They require mobility of the joints and spine, length in the muscles and coordination of the breath and body.

- Develops concentration.

- Ground through the standing leg; grow roots.

- Imagine the hip joints moving freely and easily.

- Imagine the spine lengthening.

Parkinson's/MS note: In both of the chair modifications, if a student has rigid or frozen shoulders, let the hand rest, elbow bent on the waist, and concentrate on turning the body.

Completing these postures brings a sense of achievement. Offer Uttanasana in its relaxed form, Rag Doll, as a counter-pose.

■ Extended Marichi's Pose (Utthita Marichyasana) (twisting with chair support)

Instruction

1. Place the chair facing to the right, so that you can hold the back of it.
2. Put the right foot up onto the chair seat.
3. Put the left hand on the right knee and the right hand on the right hip, or keep hold of the chair.
4. Engage the core muscles and turn to the right, towards the knee. Keep the body upright, spine long, and breathe out on the turn.

Teaching focus

- Firm standing leg, foot rooted into the ground.
- Long spine; grow tall.
- Imagine energy moving in a spiral action up through the spine.
- Turn further, even in minute amounts, on the exhale breath.

Further modifications can be offered by placing the chair against the wall:

Instruction

1. Stand with the right side to the wall and the chair in front.
2. Bring the right foot up onto the chair, and root down through the standing foot.
3. Grow tall, and turn in towards the wall.
4. Place both hands on the wall, with elbows bent, to stabilise, and breathe deeply.
5. Lengthening the spine, turn a little more into the wall on the exhale breath. Keep the shoulders open, feeling as if they are moving down and back.

■ Chair Pose (Utkatasana)

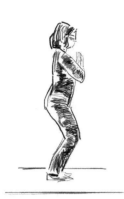 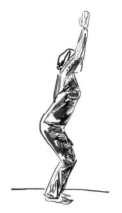 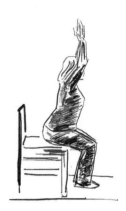

This posture will aid stability through building core strength.

Instruction

1. Stand with the feet together, and bring the palms together in prayer position.

2. Inhale, and on the exhale breath draw up the pelvic floor – Mula Bhanda. Draw in the abdominal muscles. Squeeze the knees together, working the adductors.

3. Bend the knees, keeping them pressed together, into a squatting position.

4. Progress to take the arms up above the head, push the tailbone back and bend at the hip in a semi-squat, as if you are going to sit on a chair.

5. Keep the chest lifted and try to hold the pose while taking some deep breaths.

This is a strenuous pose – it builds strength, encouraging a sense of grounding.

Teaching focus

- You are building a strong core; hold it firmly.

- Breathe long and deep.

- Feel that you are strongly rooted in the floor – connect into the feet and spread the toes.

- Only lift the arms as far as is comfortably possibly, and make allowances for shoulder injuries.

- For a variation, place a block between the knees, and squeeze the block.

Parkinson's/MS note: Those with Parkinson's and MS will have varying abilities with this posture – for some it will be far too much, and others will achieve it. You will need personal information from each individual to be able to offer this in an adapted way for them. Working with chair support will aid balance and enable leg and hip stretches where simple standing is a challenge. This gradually builds strength and confidence.

For those students who cannot stand for too long, offer a chair version.

Instruction

1. Sit on the 'sit' bones, knees together; your feet can be on a block and hands in prayer position.

2. Exhale and engage the pelvic floor – Mula Bhanda. Draw in the abdominals and squeeze the knees together.

3. Hollow the thoracic spine and lean forward slightly, as if you are going to rise from the chair.

4. Lift the arms up, if you are able.

5. Breathe deeply for four breaths.

■ Adapted versions of Wide-legged Forward Bend Pose (Prasarita Padottasana) (wide-leg rotation)

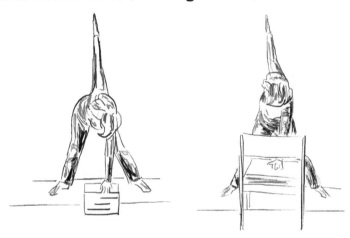

This posture can be assisted by using blocks to start with. Its wide-leg stance offers a further challenge to bring stability and energy into the legs, building a firm base.

Instruction

1. Start by placing a block or two in front of you, and stand with a wide stride so that the blocks are in front and in the middle (these may not be needed by everyone and can easily be taken away).

2. Wriggle your feet wider and place your hands on the hip joint, to bring awareness to where the bend will begin.

3. Inhale and grow tall, lengthening the spine.

4. Exhale and bend forward, as you send the tailbone back. Allow the knees to bend if they need to do so, but do not strain to keep them straight.

5. Place both hands on the block.

6. Inhale and bring one arm out to the side at shoulder height, and then rotate the body to lift the arm upright. Go only as far as is possible for you.

7. Hold and breathe.

8. Exhale, turn the body and bring the arm back to the starting position.

9. Repeat on the other side.

Teaching focus

- Encourage stable foot position and grounding, and bring awareness to the flow of Apana.

- Breathe to aid the movements.

- Encourage the turn to happen from the thoracic spine rather than the waist and hips.

- Breathe along the spine, following the gentle twisting action – imagine energy radiating outwards.

- Check that there is no hunching of the spine – add more blocks or offer a chair to keep the spine long.

■ Chair-supported version

If bending is impossible, or if the student has high blood pressure, use a chair placed in front so that the bend is not so far.

Instruction

1. Make the same preparations as before, a wide stride, this time facing the chair seat. Exhale and hinge at the hips and bend with a long spine.

2. Place both hands on the chair seat and lift one arm out to shoulder height on the inhale breath, and continue to turn the torso as far as possible. Exhale and return and repeat on the other side.

3. Place your elbows on the chair seat and lift one arm out to shoulder height on the inhale breath, and continue to turn the torso as far as possible. Exhale and return and repeat on the other side.

■ Seated rotation

Instruction

For version 1:

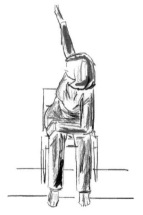

1. Sit up on the 'sit' bones with the feet parallel, knees together and inhale.

2. Exhale and bend forward from the hips and place the left forearm over the knees.

3. Lift the right arm out to shoulder height on the inhale breath, and continue to turn the torso as far as possible.

4. Exhale, and then repeat four times.

5. Repeat on the other side.

For version 2:

1. Place a pile of blocks on the floor in front of you. Adjust the height so that you can place your hands on the blocks while keeping the spine long and legs wide.

2. Sit on the chair with your legs wide, blocks in front. Inhale.

3. Exhale and bend forward from the hips and place your hands on the blocks.

4. Lift the right arm out to shoulder height on the inhale breath, and continue to turn the torso as far as possible.

5. Exhale, and then repeat four times.

6. Repeat on the other side.

■ Semi-squatting

This is a good way to strengthen the legs and knees.

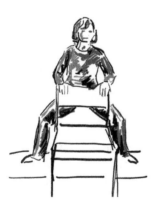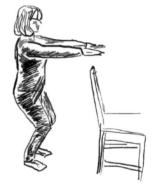

Instruction

1. With the back of the chair facing, so that it can be used if needed, stand with the feet wide apart, angled out at 45° (hold the chair if needed).

2. Keep the spine upright.

3. Engage the pelvic floor.

4. Take a gentle knee bend, directing the knees to align with the second toe. Draw up the insteps and don't let the ankles collapse.

5. Do several repeats, taking the movement deeper each time.

Teaching focus

- Good alignment of the feet and knees.
- Keep the spine as upright as possible.
- Pelvic floor engaged.

Contraindication: This posture is not suitable for a person with haemorrhoids.

◼ Feet parallel version

Instruction

1. Face the chair back with the feet parallel.
2. Engage the pelvic floor and abdominals and bend both knees and hips as if you are going to sit down, simultaneously bringing the arms forward towards the chair.
3. Let them come above the chair back.
4. Hold the posture for a slow count of ten.
5. Return to upright.
6. Repeat and build up the holding time.

◼ Transferring

Getting up and out of a chair is something that we all need to work on as we get older, so that we can build strength. This can usefully follow on from the semi-squat asanas.

Instruction

1. Sit in a chair. Practise using the pelvic floor and abdominal muscles by contracting in and up. (This is emphasised throughout the book in almost all of the practices as it is an essential factor in stability, mobility and back care.)
2. Keep your feet parallel and feel them on the floor.
3. Press them into the floor, breathe out and engage the core; lean forward, keeping the natural curve in the spine, and guide the knees over the toes, reach the arms forward, and let the crown of the head lead the movement.
4. Follow the movement through, lifting off the chair just a few inches, and hold.
5. Try to sit down slowly and control the action. The chair *is* still there.
6. Practise this often.

LYING POSTURES FOR STRENGTH AND STABILITY

Lying postures can help to strengthen the legs and spine and offer an option where standing is difficult, owing to balance, blood pressure or general weakness and balance difficulty. These asanas can follow a floor-based warm-up.

◼ Leg-raising actions

These movements are strengthening for the lower back, and need to be worked with care so that any back problems are not made worse. If in doubt, ask the student how it feels for them and work pain-free. We can use dynamic moving actions and static postures. You do not need to do all of them in one go, but select those that are suitable for the group you are working with.

Instruction

1. For bicycling, bend one knee up and then straighten it up towards the ceiling. Don't worry whether you can straighten your leg.

2. Draw in the abdominal muscles and then lower the leg slowly towards the floor, but pull it back in before you get there.

3. Using the leg in a cycling movement, do three cycles one way and three the other. (Chair versions of these can be found in on page 197)

4. Lift and lower.

5. Bend the knee and straighten the leg.

6. Hold firmly for a count of ten (hands can be used to hold the leg at first).

7. Explore whether the leg can be lowered straight, but bend if needed.

8. Lift and hold using a strap.

9. Loop the strap around the foot and use it to steady the straightening action, holding the strap like reins. Stretch the heel away, foot flexed.

10. In this position turn the toes out to turn the hip and draw an imaginary circle on the ceiling. Repeat on the other side.

11. Using the strap, and straightening the leg, place one hand on the hip, to keep the hips parallel and discourage rolling.

12. Take the straight leg out to the side. Repeat the movement in and out.

13. Do the same with the other leg.

14. Lifting both legs: if the spine is strong enough, engage the core muscles and lift both legs.

15. Hold them firm and straight for a couple of breaths.

16. Lower them in a controlled way, keeping the core muscles engaged. Bend the knees if the back is not strong enough.

This is contraindicated for some back problems.

Teaching focus

- It is important for the student to work within their own limitations, and to rest when they need to.

- Core strength.

- Muladhara chakra.

■ Bridge Pose (Setu Bhandasana or Dwi Pada Pitham)

This is important for building strength, particularly in the lower back, hamstrings, gluteus maximus and knee joints, stretching the quadriceps and opening the front of the hip joint. For promoting strength and stability we should place more emphasis on using the core muscles and less on creating an arched spine.

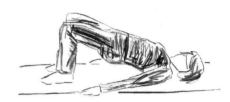

Proper alignment is essential. The feet, knees and hips should maintain parallel alignment with the feet placed near to the body, so that on lifting the hips the knees do not extend beyond the ankles. This placement needs to be checked individually. The head should be in line with the spine, supported to maintain the line of the spine, and arms with palms placed down on the floor.

The traditional breathing in this posture is to lift on an in-breath, encouraging expansion in the chest, but we can also explore the internal workings of the core muscles and diaphragm by lifting on an exhale breath.

Instruction

1. Inhale, curl the pelvis up and begin to 'peel' the spine off the floor, lifting the hips. To assist the action, press the feet into the floor and squeeze the gluteal muscles.

2. Lift as high as is possible at this time, keeping the knees parallel throughout.

3. Depending on strength and ability, hold the posture while breathing or begin to come down.

4. To return to the floor, keep awareness in the spine and lower from the top to the bottom. Connect each vertebra into the floor and roll the tailbone down last of all.

This posture can be repeated, or can be held where there is steadiness, without lifting too high.

Teaching focus

- Check alignment.
- Encourage strength in the buttocks and hamstrings.
- Keep the lift to a level that maintains steadiness.
- Strong connection to the earth through the feet, arms, shoulders and head.
- Awareness in the movement of the spine and control of the action.

Parkinson's note: Alignment will need to be done every time, as students do not always hold the information from week to week. Head placement and parallel lines are key. There may be weakness in one side of the body, which may mean the hips are not lifted equally, and the student is often unaware of this. Use gentle hand placements to encourage the movements that need addressing to attain balance.

Contraindication: If there is severe kyphosis of the spine it may not be possible to do this without discomfort.

Some knee problems may be problematic. However, each case is individual. Working with Ahimsa, and an open dialogue with the student, you can explore what may be useful and possible.

Plank (Phalankasana)

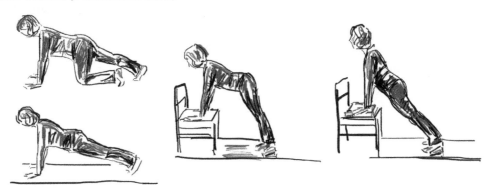

Being able to support our bodyweight is vital in enabling transition out of the chair, and up and down from the floor. This asana can help to maintain that strength and ability. Work towards Plank Pose in stages, and progress as the students get stronger. This will help when transferring from lying to sitting and to standing.

Instruction

1. Begin with simple weight-bearing postures, such as starting in Cat Pose (see page 51) as described in preliminaries, with the hands placed under the shoulders and knees under hips.

2. Transfer the weight of your body forward so the hands, arms and shoulder bear more, to become accustomed to taking weight.

3. Rock the weight back into the knees, and then repeat the action a few times more. Keep the spine in a straight horizontal line.

4. Breathe in, breathe out, and draw the abdominal muscles in and the pelvic floor up.

5. Lift the knees a little way off the floor, and try to hold.

6. Repeat four times.

7. Over the weeks, when strength is building, you can progress to taking one foot back, toes curled under, keeping the hips low and the core muscles engaged.

8. Take the other foot back taking the weight of the body for a short time, before placing the knees back on the floor.

9. Rest back into your heels with arms stretched forward in Swan Pose (see page 109).

Progress to full Plank Pose, keeping the hips low and the legs and spine aligned.

Teaching focus

- Take into account any difficulties that the individuals may have with their hands and toes. If their toes are painful or are badly affected by arthritis or spasm, they will not be able to do this.

- Allow students to find their level of ability and explore their level of strength.

- Let the students come out of the pose in their own time.

- Focus on the positive aspects that even attempting this posture brings – strength and confidence.

- Praise small achievements.

This is contraindicated for carpel tunnel.

Shoulders and upper back

Tension in the shoulders inevitably has an emotional charge. Think of all the physical expressions of emotion that refer to the shoulders – hugging, squeezing, caressing, reaching out, grasping, carrying, expressing need, depression, suppression, shock, openness, receptivity, responsibility. The shoulder and arm functions belong to the heart chakra, Anahata.

What do our shoulders say? For example, we 'shoulder responsibility', 'we carry our burdens here', we 'shoulder someone out of the way', 'put our shoulders to the wheel', 'shrug off a problem', our shoulders droop when we feel down and when we are defeated or exhausted. We protect ourselves by keeping them stiff, hunched or curled round. This physical pattern communicates something to the world about how we are feeling inside.

In Parkinson's, the posture changes, through no choice of the individual, but it will have a bearing on how they are perceived by the world. Thus it is vital to prevent or slow down the process.

These postural patterns, if held constantly, cause some muscles to harden into a chronic state and others to weaken, and those with Parkinson's or MS are then prone to injury and pain.

Posture is a challenge for those with Parkinson's and MS. Parkinson's is often characterised by a shuffling walk and stooped posture as the body loses proprioception, and a pattern of muscle weakness and spasm pulls the spine into a round-shouldered, drooping head position. Constriction in the brachial plexus and in the cervical spine may produce symptoms of tingling in the hands and numbness. The 'shoulder swing' when walking is lost as Parkinson's progresses; therefore freeing up this area is important. In MS, numbness and spasm inhibit ease of movement and stability.

Working yoga practice with conscious awareness of the aligned posture has a positive impact not only in counteracting this symptom, but also in the self-confidence and optimism that is embodied in an open upright stance. It is essential that the shoulders maintain mobility, and that correct use of the thoracic spine in yoga postures is encouraged. If you are teaching students with Parkinson's, awareness of the head, neck and upper back must be brought into all the yoga practices. It is vital to 'unglue' the shoulder blades, to release and lengthen the pectoral muscles and to bring the trapezius and rhomboids into proper tone, along with the action of the subscapularis and teres major. Of course each muscle does not work alone – so it is important to work the whole body, even if you are giving special attention to a specific area.

Warm-ups for the shoulders begin on page 43 along with some preliminary stretches for the whole body, and these should be done first.

SHOULDER-MOBILISING AWARENESS

This is a very simple action, and its efficacy relies on applying the mind and using awareness enquiry.

Instruction

1. From Mountain Pose (Tadasana) or a seated position, take all your awareness into your right arm, as if nothing else exists, just your right arm. Feel the length of your arm and the weight of your arm; experience the whole arm right to the fingertips.

2. Move it across your body to the left, lifting it with an awareness of how the muscles are working and observing any changes in the feel of your arm as you circle it around and up.

3. Slowly describe a circle with your fingertips. Be aware of the feel in the upper arm, the weight of the arm, and find the place where the action changes, as you begin to lower it, to complete the circle. Hold your full attention on every part of the journey.

4. Repeat this three times, slowly, letting the fingertips describe a bigger circle each time.

5. After working one side, pause, to allow comparison between the two sides. How does the worked arm feel? Does it feel bigger, lighter, warmer, heavier? Alive?

6. Work the other side in the same way. Pause at the end to make further comparison.

■ Swinging the shoulders

Arm stiffness is another problem for those with nervous system impediments. As the spasm and rigidity begin to take hold, it is difficult to release and soften the muscles of the shoulder girdle. Taking time to practice swinging the arms will also help the gait. I suggest beginning with backward and forward swings, letting the shoulders be as loose as possible. Swing both arms together, and try not to deliberately 'place' them. Then try cross-crawl type movements, using opposites, left, forward, right, back. Keep up encouraging comments: 'keep it really loose', 'let go', 'it doesn't matter if you aren't doing it right'.

Adding arm swings into other postures provides another opportunity to practise – try adding them to Warrior Pose 1, for example.

■ Be an elephant

I love to have the element of play and laughter in the room, and this brings awareness and a sense of release, whether the student feels it is a challenge or not.

Instruction

1. Lean forward and rest one hand on the back of a chair so that you are slightly stooped. Let the other arm just dangle. Pretend it's not your arm, that it's a puppet arm.

2. Begin to shift your body, slightly moving your hips and body, to see if you can make your arm swing without deliberately using the arm muscles.

3. Imagine the weight of the arm allowing a space in the shoulder capsule. See if you can get the arm to swing back and forth and then around and around, just by changing the movement of the body.

4. Do the same on the other side. Holding a weight such as a can of beans will help to open it up further.

◼ Pectoral stretch

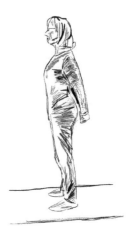

This movement is often used as a preliminary stretch for some forward-bending postures, the Warrior Poses and Cow Face Pose (Gomukhasana). The object is to stretch the pectoral muscle – it is effective if it is over-used, over-tight, pulling the shoulder forwards. This will enable the upper back to lengthen and lift.

Props can be used to help the arm spacing if mobility is limited. A resistance band, block or strap could all be useful, held behind the back.

Instruction

1. Stand in Mountain Pose (Tadasana) with feet, knees and hips parallel.

2. Clasp your hands behind your back or hold a wrist with one hand. Draw the shoulder blades together and down. Do not bow forwards or jut the chin forwards. Go only within your limitation.

3. Draw the arms down towards the floor, and then release and let go. Repeat this five times.

4. Draw down and away from the back on an inhale breath, releasing on the exhale breath. Lift the arms back and away as far as is possible; this will vary greatly from person to person.

Teaching focus

* Keep the action in the shoulder joint.

* Check individuals for chin thrusting or leaning forwards.

* Maintain a long spine.

* Encourage breath coordination.

* Encourage a little more lift on the repeats with a pain-free range.

* If standing or balance is an issue, this pose can also be done using a chair. The student would sit sideways on the chair, to enable the movement back and away, using a block, strap or band if necessary.

* Do not 'assist' a student by drawing their arms back for them.

Contraindications and modifications: Do not do this if there is pain or there has been shoulder injury. Proceed with caution, working in Ahimsa.

Parkinson's note: Hands are sometimes subject to spasm, making the ability to clasp difficult. It may be easier to hold the wrist or the sides of a block.

■ Arm angles

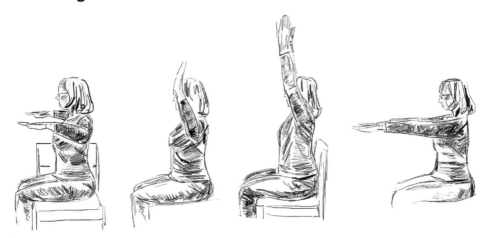

Instruction

1. Stand or sit.

2. Inhale and bring the arms up to shoulder height in parallel, palms facing down.

3. Exhaling, move the arms laterally, bending the elbows at right angles, so that the elbows are on level with the shoulders, palms down and fingers pointing forward.

4. Inhaling, and keeping the elbows in position, lift the forearms up, fingers towards the ceiling.

5. Exhale and push upwards, as if you are pushing up a sash window, arms extended.

6. Inhale as you lower your arms back to the start position.

7. Repeat four times.

■ Cow Face Pose (Gomukhasana) (arms only)

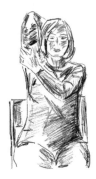 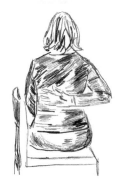 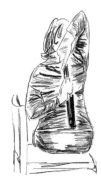

This can be practised standing or sitting. If sitting, space is needed to move the arms freely. Note that it is important to allow the student to find their own way with this, and not to manipulate, push or 'help' them physically. The shoulder joint is a shallow joint and it would be easy to dislocate in some people.

Instruction

Do this for each arm before trying the final posture:

1. Reach one arm up over the head and bend the elbow to reach back behind your head.

2. With your free hand, grip the triceps muscle and squeeze and press your way along to the elbow, as if you are helping to make the muscle longer. Do this a couple of times.

3. Wriggle the fingers of the top hand down towards the top of the spine.

4. Let go and do this on the other side.

5. With your arms behind your back, grasp hold of the forearms, near to the elbows if you are able.

6. Slide the arms from side to side (there could be considerable limitation in this action).

7. Clasp your hands behind your back. If possible, move them over to the left side of the waist, press them in against your waist, and open your shoulders further, and then move them to the other side.

8. Further exploration of the range of movement can be done by holding a strap, band or block behind your back with straight arms. Practise the side-to-side movement.

9. Practise sweeping the arm with the palm back, out to the side and round, to come up in the centre of the back.

For the full posture, have a strap and drape it over your right shoulder in preparation:

1. From Mountain Pose (Tadansana) or seated position, swing your right arm forwards and up towards the ceiling, and bend it back at the elbow to touch the base of the neck with your hand.

2. Reach the left arm forward and sweep it around to the left; turn the palm back, so that the back of the hand rests against the back of the spine. See how far the hand can come up into the middle of the back – reach up for the space between the shoulder blades.

3. Notice whether there is distortion in the upper body to achieve this. Focus the action in the shoulder; be guided by the teacher's words.

4. If your hands do not touch, feel for the strap and hold it, with both hands.

5. Creep the fingers towards each other.

6. Find the place where you can comfortably hold steady and draw the shoulders back and down, lengthening the spine; the head and neck should be upright. This can be held while it is comfortable.

7. Release, shake out the arms and then repeat on the other side.

Teaching focus

- Observe the upper back and shoulder action, and watch for any straining. Many students strive to accomplish this, and in doing so incur strains. Encourage awareness and be vigilant.

- Encourage working within personal limits and a pain-free range.

- Give permission to stop or to use props.

- Encourage the students to smile, to relax their facial muscles.

Contraindication: Shoulder injuries – some respond well while others could worsen.

■ Eagle Pose (Garudasana) (arms only)

This can be done sitting or standing, and it works the subscapularis, teres major and minor and rhomboid muscles.

Instruction

To begin:

1. Bring the palms together, elbows apart. Bring the elbows together, and press the forearms together, and move them both upwards gradually (find your personal limit), and then lower them, bringing the elbows apart. Repeat this a few times.

2. Bend the right arm, and hook the left arm underneath, pulling the elbow towards the body. Release and repeat. Do this with the other arm.

For full arm position:

3. Bend both arms and cross them over at the elbow, the left under the right, and see whether it is possible to twine the forearms and hands around to stabilise the position before attempting to lift them. Then work this with the other arm on top. This is not an easily achievable position for those with spasm and rigidity, but the preliminary stretches will be beneficial and help mobility.

Teaching focus

- Allow the whole practice to be an exploration of mobility rather than striving to achieve a perfect posture.

- Encourage students to stay within the simplest practice, and allow time to stretch there.

- Work with Ahimsa.

Parkinson's note: Spasm in the hands may be a limitation, and often full and strenuous stretching can make the tremor worse temporarily.

SUPINE SHOULDER RELEASES

A simple way to begin is to start in semi-supine, with the arms down by the sides.

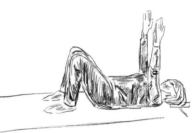

Instruction

1. Breathe in and lift your arms up and over towards the floor above the head.

2. Keep the back of the ribs on the floor to separate the shoulder action from the movement of the spine, even if it limits the shoulder action. Breathing in on the lift and lowering on the out-breath encourages coordination.

3. This movement could be done standing with your back against the wall, with the same focus into the upper back.

Teaching focus

- It is important to observe the students in action and remind them to work within their own limits.

- Check that the spine is not arching up in order to help lift the arms.

- Check the position of the head and neck, as the student might need support.

- Keep the neck long.

- Allow a little time at the end of the range to stretch into the chest and shoulder joint.

- Coordinate breathing.

The following exercise is a great way to unglue the shoulder blades and provide some ease in any tension that may be held in the trapezius. It can also be worked in a sitting position, although this will not have the same releasing effect.

■ Shoulder drops

Instruction

1. Lie in semi-supine position, with knees bent.

2. Stretch both arms up towards the ceiling, palms facing in.

3. Reach up with the right arm as if you are going to touch the ceiling, lifting the shoulder blade off the floor.

4. Let the shoulder drop back to the floor while the arm is still held up.

5. Reach with the left, and drop. Repeat five times.

6. With the arms lifted up to the ceiling, clasp your hands.

7. Push upwards and lift the outer edge of shoulder blades up off the floor and then drop back. Repeat this a few times and then progress to taking the clasped hands overhead towards the floor, only going as far as is within your capabilities.

8. For a variation, with the hands clasped and pointing to the ceiling, draw a circle 'on the ceiling' one way and then the other way.

Teaching focus

- Keep the head and neck long; support with a block.

- Encourage the action of release as the shoulder blade comes back to the floor.

■ Fish Pose (Ardha Matsyendrasana)

Students who are fit and able will be able to practise this pose as it is normally taught in a general class. It may prove difficult for those students who are unable to get to the floor and for those with a kyphotic spine. It does, however, provide a good opening stretch for the chest, and helps to counteract the rounding of the spine if it can be practised early on in diagnosis.

I describe here an adaptation, for those who can work on the floor.

■ Supported Fish Pose adaptation

This helps free the upper back and releases the shoulders. It provides a passive stretch to encourage release through the joint of the spine and shoulder.

You will need a block for under the head and/or a folded blanket for under the spine.

Instruction

For the block supported version:

1. Place the block under your back with the top of the block widthways, roughly level with the points of the shoulder blades, so that the upper back bends over the top of the block. You can also experiment with the block used longways under the spine.

2. Lie back so that the upper back is held in a gentle arch. Have the other block placed under your head to keep the neck long. More support under the head may be needed.

3. The arms can rest out to the side to open the shoulders, palms facing up.

4. Breathe in this position, taking time to let go of any held tension.

5. Remove the block or roll away, curl the legs into the chest to counter the stretch. Rock gently from side to side, if you are on your back.

Restorative variation:

1. Roll a firm blanket into a long sausage shape and place it on the floor. Sit at the bottom end and lie back so that the blanket is under the spine. This will give a gentle lift and allow the muscles either side of the spine to release. Support the head if needed.

2. Stay there and breathe easily. Relax.

Both of these are restorative postures that are meant to allow the body to find a new easier position, and give time in stillness to allow the muscle to find a new 'feel' of release.

Teaching focus

- Check that the block is in the correct place to enable a mild supported extension of the upper spine.

- Make sure that the neck is supported, particularly if there is severe contraction of the back of the neck.

- You may need to give the knee support.

- Give the student time to release in the posture and breathe.

- Heart opening – Anahata visualisations can be used.

■ Downward-facing Dog Pose (Ardho Mukha Svanasana)

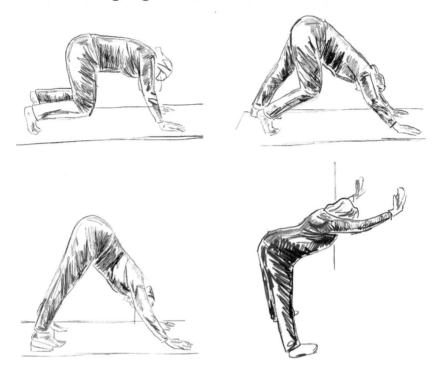

This is a great open shoulder stretch, and as it is an inverted posture, it brings blood flow into the head and shoulders. It needs to be managed and adapted if people cannot get to the floor, in which case offer the wall or a chair version (see pages 107–108).

For the most part it is a good remedial pose for frozen shoulders, depending on the level of pain. It may make some shoulder injuries worse, so individual evaluation is needed. It is useful in aiding breathing, but contraindicated for high blood pressure and glaucoma, and offers an opportunity for weight bearing to build stamina.

Instruction

Preliminaries for the floor version:

1. Have blocks to hand and possibly a wedge-shaped block and folded blanket and/or towel. Work the wrists and ankles first, with flex and extend. If there is pain in these joints or rigidity, offer a wedge-shaped block or folded blanket under the heels and wrists. Make sure that toes are able to bend and support weight.

2. Start in Cat Pose on hands and knees (see page 51), with the hands a little forward of the shoulders. Check the hand and arm position, so that the heel of the hand around the base of the thumb to the outside edge is evenly spread on the floor. Connect through all of the fingers, as if they are suctioned on to the floor. The insides of the elbows should face each other, enabling the shoulders to open.

3. Begin to lift the knees gradually off the ground, and tread the heels down alternately, to ease the hamstrings. Bring the knees back to the floor for rest time, and repeat.

4. Stay with this until you feel ready to explore the pose further.

5. When this has been worked, attempt to lift both knees together. Lift onto the balls of the feet and lower the heels gradually to the mat/support. Do not force the knees to straighten. Pay attention to the shoulders, spine and hands. Continue to let the hands be actively engaged in gripping the mat. (You may like to hold a brick-shaped block rather than have the hand flat, but make sure it won't slip on the mat.)

6. Move the body back towards the legs and create a hollow back as much as is possible.

7. Breathe gently; do not force the breath – breathing should be comfortable. This posture enables some 'draining' of the chest if it can be held with comfort.

8. Find when you need to stop from your own awareness.

9. Bring the knees back to the floor and rest with your hands resting beside your feet, shoulders dropped towards the floor.

Downward-facing Dog Pose (Ardho Mukha Svanasana), using the wall

This is the same as the half forward bend, but with the focus in the shoulders.

Instruction

1. Reach forward to put both hands on the wall, and step back, with your feet a little wider than your hips. Lengthen your tailbone back and extend your upper back. Stretch through the shoulders.

2. To come out of this pose, simply step towards the wall. An easy counter-pose could be a gentle twist from a standing, sitting or lying position to release the spine.

Teaching focus

- Encourage the extension of the upper spine and stretch through the shoulders.

- Move the posture along by encouraging a deeper stretch and giving breathing instructions.

- Caution is needed if the spine has kyphosis or severe scoliosis, or if there are shoulder injuries.

- Energy focus can be in Swadhistana and Muladhara.

This adaptation in full Downward-facing Dog Pose enables people with problems that would normally be contraindicated, such as glaucoma and high blood pressure, to experience the shoulder opening and hamstring stretching safely.

■ Downward-facing Dog Pose (Ardho Mukha Svanasana), using a chair

This enables people to bend a little further but remain standing.

Instruction

1. Stand in front of the chair.

2. Lean down and place both hands on the chair, inside of the elbows facing in.

3. Step back, feet apart, as far as possible; bend from the hips and tilt the pelvis down. Feel the stretch in the back of your legs and extend your spine.

4. Allow the neck to lengthen and continue to stretch through the shoulders and breathe into the stretch.

Teaching focus

- Visualise the joint opening and easing, imagining that there is space in the joint capsule.

- The knees can be bent if they need to be.

■ Downward-facing Dog Pose (Ardho Mukha Svanasana), seated version

Instruction

1. Sit on the chair with the wall in front of you. Pull the chair close up to the wall. Sit with the feet parallel.

2. Reach out and up, and place your hands on the wall, a little wider than your shoulders.

3. Press against the wall and lean in. Create an extension in your spine and stretch through the shoulders.

4. Walk your hands higher.

5. Stay at the end of your range and breathe. Hold for five breaths.

6. Walk your hands back down and soften your shoulders.

Parkinson's/MS note: If there is numbness or stiffness in the hands and fingers, paying attention to the positioning of the hands, the grip on the floor and bearing weight through the arms can be really helpful. If rheumatoid arthritis is present, take care to work within a pain-free range, but encourage a gentle stretch, giving permission to stop and explore personal limits.

■ Hero Pose (Virasana) (kneeling forward bend, sometimes known as Extended Swan or Extended Child's Pose, Utthita Balasana)

Instruction

1. Prepare any props – blocks and rolled towel or blanket.

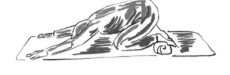

2. Beginning in Cat Pose on all fours (see page 51), place a block between your feet (or two blocks if the knee bend is limited), and roll the towel to support the ankles. Rock backwards and forwards, lowering your hips closer to the block each time.

3. Press the sit bones into the block, and begin to walk your hands forward, keeping your spine long and opening up your shoulder joint.

4. Maintain length through from your tailbone to the crown of your head.

5. Keep your head low – supporting the head on a block assists in maintaining a long neck.

6. Hold the stretch for as long as you feel comfortable. Breathe normally.

7. Walk your hands back in and lift yourself out of the posture.

8. Unfold your legs and sit on the block with knees bent, easing out any parts that need it.

Teaching focus

- Check that the knees and ankles are supported if there is any limitation.
- Encourage working within personal limitation.
- Ahimsa – make sure that students are working with comfort and are not forcing the pose.
- Focus on the shoulder joint and visualising openness and release.

Contraindication: Inflamed joints, knee ligament problems and varicose veins.

■ Hero Pose (Virasana), chair version

As some students may be severely limited through the hips and knees, this version using two chairs may be more suitable. Use two chairs facing each other.

Instruction

1. Sit on one chair with the other chair placed in front of your knees.

2. Bend from the hips and, lengthening the tailbone, reach forward to hold the chair in front.

3. Walk your hands forward, keeping the spine long.

4. Keep your head low, neck long and spine lengthening.

5. Hold and breathe normally.

6. To return, walk your hands in and lift your spine.

7. Ease and release. Return to an upright position.

■ Thread the needle

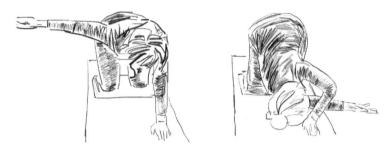

I tend to call this the 'Feeling for Something Under the Sofa' Pose. I am not sure from whence this movement derives, but from my own experience it manages to stretch the muscles of the musculotendinous cuff in an efficient way.

Instruction

1. Begin in Cat Pose (see page 51), with the hands placed under the shoulders on the mat.

2. Lift the right arm out to the side, to shoulder height, palm facing down.

3. Bring your arm down and move the hand through the arch made by the left arm and the body, sliding the back of your hand on the floor. Look over your left arm to keep your spine long.

4. Bend your left elbow. Your right shoulder and the side of your head should come to the floor as you reach the right arm further along the floor.

5. Withdraw your right arm slowly, and repeat this on the other side.

6. Sit up and ease out the shoulders afterwards.

Teaching focus

• Be aware of tension held in the armpit area and around the shoulder blades.

■ Thread the needle, wall version

Instruction

1. Stand close to the wall, about 40 cm or so away. Place your hands on the wall.

2. Lift the right arm out to the side and then slide the back of the hand under the left arm arch and along the wall.

3. Connect your right shoulder to the wall and the side of your head, and inch your hand a little further.

4. Return and go on the other side.

This, and Hugs (see page 44), will stretch the area similarly, but without the weight of the body that working on the floor provides, although this may be a useful option for students who are unable to be on the floor.

■ Belly Twist Pose
(Jathara Parivartanasana) (reclined twist variation)

There are a few different ways to approach this posture. This method pays particular attention to the upper back and the relationship between the shoulders, thoracic spine and breastbone.

This is a floor pose, but a similar action can be facilitated from a seated position, if there is difficulty in transferring to and from the floor.

This stretch gives an opportunity to mobilise the thoracic spine and to stretch the pectoral muscles.

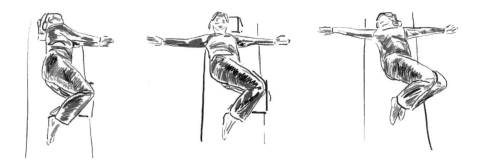

Instruction

1. Lie on your side with the spine straight, head supported on a block so that the neck is in line with the spine and not drooping; add further support where necessary, and have the knees bent. It may take a little adjustment to get into the correct position, but this will enable you to work specifically in the upper back.

2. Have the arms stretched forwards at shoulder height on the floor, palms together.

3. Lift the top arm up towards the ceiling; this arm position should remain in place, in relation to the breastbone and upper back.

4. Engage the pelvic floor and core muscles and squeeze the knees together – a block between the knees can help.

5. Inhale as you turn from the breastbone and let the spine turn, to lower the top arm towards the floor, without over-extending at the shoulder joint.

6. Hold the posture and breathe normally.

7. On an exhale, and with the knees stable and keeping the core muscles engaged, return the body to the starting position.

8. Repeat this four times and then allow a pause in the stretch position, to feel into the posture.

9. Repeat on the other side.

Teaching focus

- Check the starting posture for alignment – have supports in place.

- Encourage the turn from the breastbone, and keep the shoulder action steady without strain.

- Breathe into the stretch.

- Encourage release in the pectoral area, enjoy the open chest, open heart feeling. Breathe here.

- Heart chakra.

- Vyana vayu.

- Feel the stretch across the upper chest.

Parkinson's note: Many people with Parkinson's will be challenged by this movement, but most will be able to get somewhere and will feel the benefits. Some spinal problems may be contraindicated. You may have to physically help people to lie in an aligned position. Guide by words and minimal hand support, with permission. This movement helps frozen shoulders, but the student should work to their own limits and practise regularly.

▉ Belly Twist Pose (Jathara Parivartanasana), chair variation

Instruction

1. Sit sideways on the chair with the knees together, and engage the pelvic floor and abdominals. Sit up on the 'sit' bones – grow tall.

2. Stretch the arms out in front at shoulder height, palms together.

3. Turning away from the back of the chair, open your arms out. Stay connected to the 'sit' bones, squeeze the knees together and feel that the breastbone turns. Let your arms open out but do not over-stretch.

4. To help focus the twist, lightly touch the breastbone with the fingertips, keeping the elbow up.

This chair version is less effective and a little harder as students do not have the support of a flat surface to support the spine.

■ Drawing a circle

You can add a further exploration of shoulder mobility by moving into 'drawing a circle', to encourage a full rotation at the shoulder.

Instruction

1. From the supine twist start position, and with arms forward at shoulder height, hands over each other, imagine that you are going to draw a circle with your top arm.

2. As you inhale, begin to bring the arm forwards and up, trailing the fingers along the floor.

3. Continue the arm circle above your head and then begin to breathe out as you complete the circle by taking your arm down to the back, and then across the hip and back to the start.

4. Explore whether you can keep your fingers on the floor.

5. Repeat three times and then try circling in the other direction, before repeating the whole thing with the other arm.

Teaching focus

- Explore the range of movement that the student can easily access.

- Check that the body is kept steady, and only the upper back turns.

- Do not force the hand to the floor; rather, allow the stretch and incremental progress.

This movement can help with a frozen shoulder, but may be limited if it is in an acute state. Try placing the top hand on the waist and then let the hand drop to the floor, to the back of the waist, and tiptoe the fingers away from the back.

Hips and pelvis

Strengthening and mobilising the lower body

Because walking and balancing pose a challenge for those with MS and Parkinson's, there can often be feelings of limited freedom, fear of dependency, of 'stepping into the future'. The hips and pelvis are the power house of the body, so when things are 'not right', we can feel disempowered and weak.

The muscles of the pelvic floor provide a support for the internal organs and a root of strength for the tailbone and spine. When holding oneself steady, and when walking and balancing become a challenge, core strength is essential. When planning Yoga Therapy practices, we have to consider that other conditions are likely to be present, such as haemorrhoids, constipation, irritable bowel syndrome or uterine prolapse.

For hip-focused asanas, use preliminary warm-ups such as some of the standing postures, Cat Pose extend and curl and hip circles, etc. (see page 51–52). Promote an active core and support Apana through awareness of grounding and good alignment, as detailed in the section on posture and the spine (see page 58). All of the standing postures, Mountain Pose (Tadasana), Warrior Pose 1 (Virabhadrasana) and balances will help to strengthen the spine, legs and feet (see pages 78, 81 and 139).

■ Sacral easing

Instruction

1. Lying with both legs straight, push the right leg away as if you are making it longer than the left, and then hitch it up as if making it shorter while simultaneously lengthening the left leg. Repeat this a few times on each side.

2. Walk the heels to the right and then to the left, while keeping the rest of the body straight. These moves will begin to stretch the lower back a little. Don't do this if it is at all painful.

Teaching focus

- Imagine creating space in the hip joint and sacroiliac joint.

WORKING IN SEMI-SUPINE

■ Hip releasing, 'tracking the heel'

In a semi-supine position, support the head to keep the neck aligned. This move is strengthening for the quads and uses the hip rotators and gluteals. It will help the teacher to identify imbalances in the hip rotators and adductors.

Instruction

1. With both knees bent, draw the right knee into the chest, holding firmly.

2. Leading with the heel, slowly slide the left leg down along the mat; try to keep the heel tracking in a straight line and do not let the knee drift inwards. Lengthen the leg and stretch.

3. Carefully begin to bend the knee and draw it back in a straight line. Repeat three times and then work the other side.

Teaching focus

- Observe the knee action carefully. A gentle touch to the side of the knee to direct the movement is all that is needed to help the student realign.

- Point out all of the action points. Deep bend the hip and knee on the held knee as well as exercising control of the straightening leg. Stretched hamstrings and Achilles tendon.

- Keep the upper body relaxed if possible.

Parkinson's/MS note: Offer a strap for the bent knee if it is needed. This will depend on the rigidity of the spine. Cramping often happens in any held stretches.

◼ Happy Baby Pose (Ananda Balasana)

Instruction

1. Lie on the mat in semi-supine.

2. Prepare for this posture by drawing each leg up onto the chest. Do this three times.

3. With the right knee drawn towards the chest, use the right hand to guide the knee towards the armpit.

4. Repeat this three times and then do the same using the other leg.

5. Draw both knees up onto the chest.

6. Part the knees and lift the feet up towards the ceiling so that the knee joint is a right angle.

7. Bring your arms to the inside of your legs and reach up to place the palms of the hands on to the soles of the feet.

8. Pull the knees down towards the outside of the armpit.

9. Release the pressure and then pull again.

10. Replace both feet back on the ground.

Teaching focus

- Deep bend in the hip, stretch through the lower back and gluteal muscles.

- Muladhara chakra.
- Some may need two straps around the feet, to assist in this posture.

■ Sciatic stretch, a 'Figure 4'

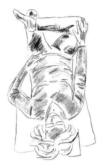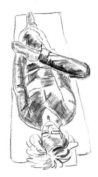

This posture requires some agility. It is hard for those with rigidity, but can ease sciatic and hip tightness. It can often result in a tangle of arms and legs, so it is worth demonstrating first.

Instruction

1. Lie in semi-supine and cross the right foot over the left knee, allowing the right knee to open out to the side as far as possible.
2. Place the right hand on the right knee and gently press it away.
3. Reach under the right leg with the right hand, and take hold of the left thigh, behind the left knee. Reach around the left leg with the left hand and hold the left thigh behind the knee. Both hands will be behind the left knee.
4. Pick the left foot off the floor and draw the leg closer if possible. Repeat on the other side.
5. Replace both feet on the floor.

Teaching focus

- Improves hip flexibility.
- Relieving sciatica.
- Fun! It's attempting the posture that counts.

Parkinson's/MS note: Working this posture requires attention and orderly thinking, and a challenge to the brain-body messaging system, so it is good to give clear instructions in a logical, step-by-step way.

■ Bridge Pose (Setu Bhandasana or Dwi Pada Pitham)

This is one of our major therapeutic postures, as there are so many benefits in practice.

This posture strengthens the lower back, knees and back of the legs, toning the gluteal muscles and stretching the quadriceps. Thus, it strengthens the back of the body while stretching the front. It opens the hip joint at the front, stretches the pectoral muscles and opens the chest. To do it we have to control our actions and increase our awareness and connection into the spine.

◼ Pelvic tilt

We can begin by encouraging the tilting action of the pelvis that instigates the movement. In itself the pelvic curl is useful in easing stiffness in the lower back.

Instruction

1. Lie in semi-supine, neck supported where required, arms down by the sides of the body.

2. Draw up the pelvic floor and engage the abdominals.

3. Press the waist into the floor and lift the tailbone off. Tilt the pelvis up, pubic bone towards the head.

4. Release and roll the tailbone down.

5. Curl up, breathe out, roll down, breathe in.

6. Use rhythmic breathing and movement. Feel an easing action in the lower back.

◼ Full Bridge Pose

Instruction

1. Proper alignment is essential. The feet, knees and hips should maintain parallel alignment, with the feet placed near to the body, so that on lifting the hips, the knees do not extend beyond the ankles. The head should be in line with the spine and supported if necessary, to maintain that line. The arms are placed palms down on the floor.

2. Traditional breathing in this posture is to lift, on an in-breath, encouraging expansion in the chest, but we can also explore the internal workings of core muscles and diaphragm by lifting on an exhale breath.

3. Inhaling, begin with the pelvic tilt and begin to 'peel' the spine off the floor as you lift the hips. To assist the action, press the feet into the floor and squeeze the gluteal muscles. Lift as high as is possible today, keeping the knees parallel throughout.

4. Depending on strength and ability, hold for a couple of breaths or begin to come down immediately.

5. To return to the floor, keep awareness in the spine and lower the spine onto the floor from the top to the bottom, connecting each vertebrae into the floor and rolling the tailbone down last of all.

This posture can be repeated, or held, where there is steadiness.

Teaching focus

- Check alignment.
- Encourage strength in the buttocks and hamstrings.
- Encourage lift.
- Lift the breastbone and breathe into the heart, Anahata focus.
- Strong connection with the earth through the feet, arms, shoulders and head.
- Awareness in the movement of the spine and control of the action.
- Talk to your spine – ease out, roll softly, enjoy the feel of the floor.

Parkinson's note: Alignment will need to be done every time, as students do not always hold the information from week to week. Head placement and parallel lines are key. There may be weakness in one side of the body, which may mean the hips are not lifted equally, and the student is often unaware of this. Use gentle hand placements to encourage the movements that need addressing to attain balance. Bridge Pose has many variations, most of which will be beyond the strength of the average person with Parkinson's, but the addition of arm lifting is a useful shoulder opener. This can be used with coordination, inhaling, lifting the hips, lifting the arms overhead. In some people, the shape of the upper spine may hinder the movement.

Contraindication: If there is severe kyphosis of the spine, it may not be possible to do this without discomfort. Some knee problems may be problematic. However, each case is individual, and working with Ahimsa, in an open dialogue with the student, explore what may be useful and possible. It is possible to move into the restorative element and offer a bolster to support the hips.

GENTLE HIP OPENERS IN THE 'ON THE SIDE' POSITION

■ Kick round and down

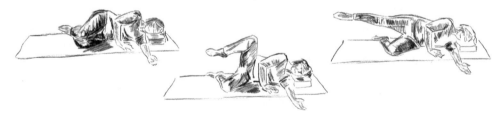

This is a good warm-up and would be a good preliminary for 'on the side' postures.

Instruction

1. Lie on your side with the spine straight and knees bent, lower arm stretched out and the other used to steady the position, head supported by blocks, to keep the line of the spine.

2. Lift the knee up in front and then circle up and out from the hip, and then straighten the leg down and pull it back up to the start.

3. Do four of these kicks and then circle the hip the other way.

4. Repeat on the other side.

◼ Lift the lid and lower

This opening and closing movement for the hips can be worked from different positions with slightly differing degrees of difficulty, but the variations enable us to place them in a sequence of postures to give flow to the class.

Instruction

1. From the same position as 'Kick round and down', lie on your side with the spine straight and knees bent, have the lower arm stretched out and the other used to steady your position, the head supported by blocks, to keep the line of the spine.

1. Keeping the feet together, lift the top knee up as far as possible, squeezing the gluteals and hip rotators.

2. Draw the knees together. This makes an opening and close movement, like 'lift the lid', 'close the lid'.

3. Roll over and work the other side.

Teaching focus

*   Check that the student is in the correct aligned position.

*   Check the head/neck position and support where needed. •

*   Engage the core muscles to steady the body so that only the hip is moving.

*   Work slowly and steadily.

Parkinson's/MS note: Students may be unable to manage stillness or accurately get themselves into an aligned position without help. Allow them to work within their own 'frame', if necessary, and look for their own alignment within their positioning. A common problem is that, without a degree of strength and control, the hips roll. Stand behind the student and use your lower leg against their hips to steady and prevent rolling. Or kneel behind them and support with your hands. A similar movement for the hips from the semi-supine position can be offered as an alternative, parting the knees, opening them as wide as is comfortable and then bringing them back together.

This movement can also be done from a sitting position, which is a little harder:

Instruction

1. Sit on a block with knees comfortably bent and core muscles engaged, hands placed on the floor for support.

2. Let one knee open out to the side, and then slowly bring it back.

3. Do this four times and then repeat on the other side.

■ Side leg lifts

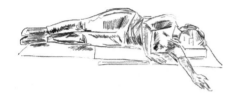 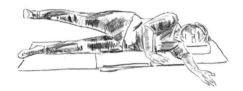

This strengthens the gluteals, abductors and adductors, as well as the core muscles used to stabilise the position.

Instruction

1. Begin by lying on the side, aligned with the back straight and knees bent, head supported by a block, and top arm used to steady the position.

2. Engage the core muscles and straighten the top leg, while keeping the body steady. Try not to roll forward or back, and stretch the heel away.

3. Relax the ankle a little so that the foot is in a comfortable position; the toes can be turned in slightly to help alignment of the knee.

4. Lift the leg up as far as is possible, and then lower. Repeat four times and then roll over to work the other side.

Teaching focus

*   This posture offers an opportunity to practise balance and core stability.

*   Check alignment and any support.

*   Engage the pelvic floor and core.

*   Work with individuals. Stand behind the student and check for rolling back. You can help with steadiness by placing your lower leg against the back of the student, to let them gain a sense of being in the right place, and see if they can manage to hold it.

*   Check that the knee doesn't turn out.

*   This can feel like a quite strenuous activity for some people, so allow a rest afterwards.

*   Progress in this posture can be made by holding for a little longer in the leg-raised position. Lifting the other leg up to meet the raised leg might be possible with practice.

SITTING POSTURES FOR HIP OPENING

Good seated posture is essential, whether on the floor or on a chair. With both of these groups of students, sitting well is as important as the standing posture. Students with Parkinson's and MS have very different capabilities and strengths, and many are unable to stand for long periods. They may tire easily or experience balance difficulties, muscle spasm or numbness, and some may find it difficult to transfer from the floor to chair or vice versa.

Practise sitting in Staff Pose (Dandasana) (see page 60), to begin to build strength.

Because of the changes in the spine either due to the disease process or ageing, sitting on the floor usually needs support. This will depend on the flexibility of the hips, tightness of the hamstrings and lower back, and the strength of the individual to hold themselves upright while sitting. Blocks are invaluable. Most people need at least one, while others may need two. More than this, and a chair may offer better support.

Being able to sit up onto the 'sit' bones, the ischia, is of primary importance, and to be able to sense the 'feel' of that position is included in every seated position, as it enables the spine to lift and the chest to open. Another block or rolled blanket may be needed to support under the knees, if the hamstrings are too tight for the legs to be straight.

■ Chair work

Attention needs to be paid to sitting well in a chair, as in this position we will be offering breathing as well as a variety of adapted postures. It is essential to sit up on the 'sit' bones, to be able to feel the feet on the floor and so establish a sturdy base. A block can be placed under the feet to help if the chair is not quite the right height. If the student is unable to sit comfortably this way, cushions can be placed to support the back. Any slumping back will inhibit breathing and constrict the chest.

■ Cross-legged positions

Sitting in a cross-legged position is used in many yoga practices, but it can be challenging where people have rigidity or numbness. Practising can help relieve some of the stiffness and ease out tight hips. Do not look for the 'perfect' posture, but let people find their own 'perfection', working to whatever is possible on the day. Offer props to support the hip/knee position – a block, cushions or rolled blankets all help with this.

What is possible? You never know till you try.

You may need to explore the possibilities of cross-legged positions fairly early on in group sessions. Can people sit on the floor? For legs-outstretched postures, offer two chairs, so that legs can be extended and the problem of transferring to and from the floor is bypassed.

Instruction

1. Experiment with an easy cross-legged pose to start with, seated on a block. If the knees are more up than down, use support near to the hip joint. Just a moment or two in this position is a stretch enough for some people.

2. Look carefully at which leg is forward, and try swapping them over.

3. Work further by pressing the knee away while leaning over the other leg.

These are good to work before Head-to-Knee Forward Bend (Janu Sirsasana).

Teaching focus

- Check that the student is sitting up on the 'sit' bones.

- The spine should be upright.

- Knees are allowed to open out and down.

- Work into the posture by placing one hand on the knee that is higher, easing it down gently.

- Do *not* force, in any way.

- Check for any arthritis of the hip, or if there has been hip replacement.

- If being on the floor or sitting cross-legged is impossible, work from a chair. Still sitting upright on the 'sit' bones, bring the right foot up to rest on the left knee, dropping the right knee out to the side. If there is any 'give' in this movement, place your hand on the right knee and press gently as if encouraging it to ease down. Do not force.

Many of the yoga postures in this section can be adapted for the chair (see page 184).

■ Warms-ups for forward fold: back and forth and rowing

Instruction

1. Sit on a block, with legs stretched forward, knees supported if needed.

2. Lift your arms forward to shoulder height, parallel with the floor. Engage the core, lean back a little way and then ease forward, hinging from the hip, while lengthening the spine and breathing out.

3. Lean back, breathing in. A block could be held to give steadiness.

4. This can be extended into a 'rowing' action. Draw the arms in as you lean back, as if pulling on oars, and then stretch up and over on the forward bend.

5. Connect this action to rhythmic breathing: engage the pelvic floor, exhale on leaning back, inhale on lifting your arms up, exhale extending over the legs, inhale returning upright.

■ Seated Forward Bend (Paschimottanasana)

If there are any spinal problems that may be contraindicated, such as an acute prolapse disc, degeneration or osteoporosis, a block should be offered to sit on, and support under the knees.

Instruction

1. Start as in the preliminary stretch (see previous page), engage the core, ease the back, and raise the arms above.

2. Lift up out of the pelvis and lengthen the spine. Imagine reaching for a trapeze bar, just above your head.

3. Move from the hips, and keep lengthening the spine in the forward bend over the legs. Let your arms come to rest somewhere on the legs or feet.

4. Come out of the pose by releasing softly over the legs; let the arms trail along the floor and feel as if you are coming out of the bend by placing one vertebrae on top of another.

Teaching focus

- Breathe into the stretch along the back of the body.

- Imagine the spine lengthening, and direct the crown of the head towards the toes.

- Check that the spine is not over-arched or the neck compressed.

- Imagine a line down the front of the body, and keep it long.

- Let the shoulders relax and soften.

- Allow the knees to bend.

- Breathe light into Swadisthana chakra.

- Visualise moving deeper into the stretch.

- Offer a simple back bend counter-pose.

- Don't let the students struggle with the goal of catching hold of their toes, or to try to put their head on their knees. When a bend that is within their own range is attained, encourage breathing and lengthening.

- Where there are arm-raising movements, it is important to take into account the shape of the spine, shoulder injuries or frozen shoulder conditions. In an effort to extend their arms above, students will often facilitate this action by over-arching the spine and neck, in an attempt to create a feeling of lift, when what is actually happening is a distortion. This is harmful if repeated often, and can cause strain in the spine and in the shoulders. Make sure that the movement is actioned from the correct joint and the shoulder extension is not forced but kept within mobility range.

Parkinson's/MS note: It is helpful to be hands-on and encourage an upright spine to allow the student to feel the difference, to 'know' their own capabilities and to identify what needs to change and how to action that change. Placing a hand lightly on part of the back to encourage length and lift will give guidance to enable the student to respond. The ability to 'do' the posture is almost irrelevant, as it is the enquiry into the body that will start to bring the biggest benefits. Give encouragement, however small the improvement might be.

■ Seated Forward Bend (Paschimottanasa), with a strap

Using a strap can greatly improve alignment and enable a more focused stretch. This will accommodate the limitations of tight hamstrings and stiffness in the spine.

Instruction

1. Sitting on a block, connect through the 'sit' bones.

2. Loop the strap around the soles of the feet and hold the strap like reins.

3. Lift the trunk up, engage the pelvic floor and lengthen the spine, as you breathe out.

4. Use the straps to pull yourself forwards, while keeping the spine long; this keeps the movement in the legs and hips, and discourages the temptation to round the spine.

5. The posture can be held while breathing and releasing a little more on the out-breath.

6. Release and come back, counter-pose with an easy back bend.

Teaching focus

- Look out for too much tension in trying to pull on the strap.

- Encourage the shoulders to stay down.

■ Bound Angle Pose (Cobbler Pose) (Bhadakonasana)

As a teacher for these specific groups of students, we have to let go of the picture of the perfect posture. We will all have books with someone modelling a beautiful upright spine and bent knees resting on the ground in this posture. It is unlikely that you will see this in your group, but this should not deter you from offering this pose. Be ready with plenty of support materials, blocks, bolsters and blankets.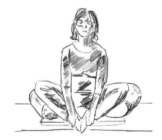

Instruction

1. Sit upright on the 'sit' bones; pay attention to lengthening the spine and feel the ground under the 'sit' bones.

2. Bring your feet together and let your knees move apart. Place the support near to the hip joint so that you can allow time for releasing. Press gently along the length of the thigh from hip to knee, but don't force it. Use the pressure as a massage, to encourage the muscle to soften and lengthen.

3. You can try a little 'butterfly' action, moving the knees up and down, and then relax back onto the supports.

4. Bring the knees back together.

5. Slide your legs straight and rub alongside the knees.

Teaching focus

- Hip release.
- Stretching the adductors.
- Being kind to oneself, acceptance.
- Finding personal limits.
- Be willing to yield.

◼ Wide-seated Forward Bend Pose (Upavista Konasana) (legs-apart stretch sequence)

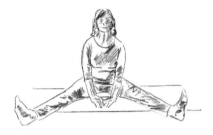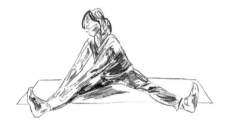

Rather than using this as a static posture, this is a set of bends that enable the adductor muscles to stretch and the hips to open.

Instruction

1. Sit up on the block, legs apart, and feel into the 'sit' bones; the legs can remain bent.
2. Engage the core and, within your own limits, turn your body to the right leg, breathe in and lean back.
3. Stretch your arms up and then exhale, bending from the hips to fold over the right leg, as far as is possible without straining.
4. Release almost immediately and return to the sitting-up position. Repeat to the left side.
5. Facing front, breathe in, lean back, stretch your arms up and lift the ribcage.
6. Bend forward and breathe out, taking one hand to each foot/knee/shin/thigh.
7. Bring the legs back together and follow with a Seated Forward Bend (Paschimottanasana). This sequence can be repeated a few times.

From this same legs-apart position, a number of variations can be done, all of which encourage strength through the torso, good positioning of the spine and shoulders, and engagement of the pelvic floor and abdominals. These serve to improve overall strength and stability. Some of these variations are:

1. From sitting upright, gently twist, to the right, keeping the body upright and shoulders level. Take your hands to the floor to your right and bend, as if you are going to put your head on the floor. Return and go to the left.

2. Another option would be to lift the arms in an outstretched position at shoulder height, with palms together above the head, parallel in front, or holding a block. Turn the torso to the left and then right.

3. A side bend preliminary could be brought in. Start with the hand on the floor to each side. Lift one arm up and bend to the other side, taking the lifted arm as far over as you can. Repeat on the other side.

4. Relax and ease out the knees, before moving into an easy back bend counter-pose.

Teaching focus

- Allow the student to find the leg width that is comfortable for them – opening too wide is a strain on the gracilis and sartorius.

- Keep connecting through the 'sit' bones.

- Muladhara and Swadhistana chakra awareness.

- Check the foot and knee position – the knee should stay on top and not roll in.

■ Easy back-bend counter-pose

Instruction

1. From the seated position, rest back on straight arms. Take a breath in and arch the back, opening the chest and lifting the breastbone up.

2. Support the neck and head by tucking the chin in slightly to engage the sternocleidomastoid. Do not let the head just loll backwards.

3. Round the spine, dropping the head forward to release the neck.

4. Move from one position to the other, or, if you have more stamina and strength, hold with breathing for four or five breaths.

Teaching focus

- Bring awareness through the whole of the spine, rooting down through the tailbone.

- Anahata awareness.

- Shoulders staying open.

CHAIR ADAPTATIONS FOR SITTING FORWARD BENDS

If the students are not able to easily transfer up and down from the floor, there are some options for bending from the chair. Blocks can be placed under the feet for those who find it difficult to connect fully with the feet on the floor.

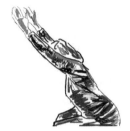 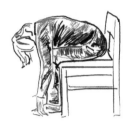

■ Simple chair bend

Instruction

1. Sit up in the chair with feet parallel on the floor. On an in-breath lift the arms and reach up, keeping the spine long.

2. Fold forward from the hip joint until the body is resting on the legs or as near as possible, and lower the arms and hands to the feet.

3. Return to upright by working the upper back by lifting the arms first on an in-breath and stretching forward. Come all the way up, arms stretched, and then lower the arms. If you are unable to lift your arms easily, return in a relaxed way, with arms soft.

4. Progress the asana by sitting towards the front of the chair, with feet parallel. Extend one leg, sliding the foot along the floor. Starting with both hands placed on the thigh, slide them down to the extent of your own range, stretching the hamstrings. Or extend the arms upwards and stretch over the straight leg, or modify this with the knee bent.

5. Repeat on the other side.

Seated Forward Bend (Paschimottanasana) from the chair is the same as chair Standing Forward Bend (Uttanasana) for those who cannot transfer from the floor. Although this does not give the same leg stretch, it will assist in keeping the spine flexible and help with muscle rigidity.

Instruction

1. With the feet parallel and placed on blocks (if that helps with the feet feeling grounded), connect into the 'sit' bones and grow tall.

2. Lift the arms in parallel, to lift the torso and lengthen the spine.

3. As you exhale, bend forward from the hips. Move into the bend slowly, going all the way down, hands to feet, or as far as they will go.

4. Soften the shoulders and keep the breathing steady.

5. You can lift out in a dynamic way, stretching the arms forwards first before lifting the spine all the way up. Or in a soft relaxed way, allowing the spine to come up vertebra by vertebra.

This asana can be made more strenuous by working more slowly and stopping halfway with the spine and arms horizontal with the floor, if the student can hold it. You can do this on both going into the bend and coming out.

A chair version of Seated Forward Bend (Paschimottanasana) can be offered with two chairs, as long as balance can be maintained. This is suitable for those who find transferring to the floor too hard, but is best with individual guidance and attention.

With both legs up on the chair in front, the student can be guided into the forward fold as directed for the floor. Two chairs can also be used as an adaptation for the one leg stretch, by simply putting one leg up on the chair in front to stretch over.

■ Sitting dynamic bend

Instruction

1. Sit up on the 'sit' bones, with legs and feet parallel.

2. Starting with the arms down by your sides, begin to breathe in and sweep them out to the sides as you lift them up, parallel.

3. Bend forward, extending and lengthening the spine, and keep the line of the arms and spine for as long as possible. Let the arms drop in a relaxed position down towards the feet. Let go.

4. Hold for a couple of shallow breaths and then breathe out, and prepare to lift the arms and spine on the inhale.

5. Stretch the arms forward parallel with the floor, press your feet into the floor and lift the spine.

6. Lower your arms out to the sides on the out-breath.

7. Repeat three times.

8. Keep this moving, so that it is a dynamic, warming, stimulating, energising flow.

■ Legs-apart forward bend, twist chair version

This is a sequence of movements that will work the spine, shoulders and the hips, and is a useful warm-up for further twisting and bending postures.

Instruction

1. Sit on the chair with the knees and feet wide, and sit up on the 'sit' bones.

2. Place the right elbow on the right knee and drop the left hand to the right ankle.

3. Sweep the left hand out and up, turning the body and shoulders on an in-breath. Breathe out and return to the start. Repeat five times on each side.

4. Turn towards the right knee, lean back, breathe in, stretch up, lift and lengthen the spine as you bend from the hip over the right thigh.

5. There are then a couple of options depending on your strength: keep the stretched-out long spine position and hold it for a couple of breaths, or immediately release over the legs, hands down onto the floor, before lifting out and coming back up.

6. All this should be repeated over the other leg.

7. From this wide-leg position, you can also do the side bend Revolved Head-to-Knee Pose (Parivrtta Janu Sirsasana): Turning the shoulders to point the right shoulder at the right knee, lift both arms, palms facing each other, or the right hand holding the left wrist, and extend over the right thigh. Keep both 'sit' bones on the chair and ease as far into the side stretch as possible. Return in a controlled way, lifting away and up. Repeat on the other side.

Teaching focus

- The action of the spine, lengthening the trunk, toning the obliques and latissimus dorsi.

- Breathing in coordination.

- Working within personal limits.

- Keeping connection with the ground.

- Manipura chakra.

◼ Head-to-Knee Pose (Janu Sirsasana) (seated one-leg bend)

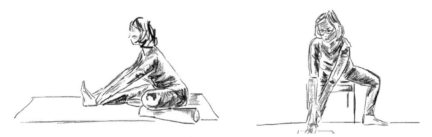

To enable a correct upright seated position and without forcing the hip, use supporting blocks and/or folded blankets; a strap may be helpful around the foot.

Instruction

1. First, prepare: with one leg in front, bend the other knee and rock it out to the side, taking care to move the whole leg from the hip and not to just force the knee down. Take time for the body to get used to this position, and wait for the joint to ease. (In older students, it is good to be kind to the joints, to give them time to release.)

2. Gently press the hand down along the thigh, and stroke down with medium pressure along the muscle from hip to knee.

3. When the outward limit of the move is found, adjust the support. This means keeping the spine upright and placing the required number of blocks in place to support the leg near the hip joint, not directly under the knee. You can build an angle from two blocks, or use a rolled blanket or bolster. When this is in place, the bent leg can rest against the support and release a little more. The straight leg may also need supporting behind the knee.

4. From this supported position you can progress to the forward bend part of the asana. Lengthen the spine upwards and lift the arms in parallel, and hinge forward over the leg, from the hip joint.

5. Let the hands come down onto the leg wherever they can, but do not try to touch the toe.

6. To return, release the stretch, soften the posture and bring the spine upright, or use the more dynamic method, extending the arms forwards, and lift the arms and spine.

This is a complex posture for the average student with Parkinson's, but these postures offer opportunities to challenge the nerve pathways and for awareness and coordination.

Teaching focus

*   Good seated posture, core engaged.

*   Encourage hip releasing by using breath, and visualising softness, freedom and space within the joint.

*   Stretching into hamstrings and spine.

*   Bring awareness into Swadhistana chakra.

■ Head-to-Knee Pose (Janu Sirsasana), with a strap

As with Seated Forward Bend (Paschimottanasana), a greater feeling of stretch and alignment is found using a strap.

Instruction

1. Sit in Staff Pose (Dandasana), on a block if needed and sitting up on the 'sit' bones. Place the strap around the sole of the foot. Leave it ready to hold, when the bent knee is in position and supported.

2. Hold the strap and ease forward with a long straight spine, encouraging the stretch to come from the hip and leg rather than the spine.

3. Deepen the posture by using the breath and making very gradual changes.

4. Release and repeat on the other side.

Teaching focus

- Check for over-stretching and tension in pulling the strap.
- Check for shoulder tension.

■ Head-to-Knee Pose (Janu Sirsasana), with a chair

There are several options to consider, depending on the student's mobility:

Instruction

1. Sitting towards the front of the chair, extend one leg (this can be supported with a block). The other leg can remain, knee bent and foot on the floor. The forward bend can then be worked over the straight leg, with or without a strap.

2. With one leg stretched out straight, let the bent leg turn out from the hip, so that the outside edge of the foot rests on the floor (or block). Lengthen the spine and bend over the straight leg.

3. Using two chairs, one placed in front of the other, lift one leg up onto the chair in front, and bend forward over the extended leg.

Teaching focus

- Sitting well.
- Check for safety and avoiding strain.

■ Revolved Side Angle Pose (Parivrtta Janu Sirsasana) (one-leg side bend)

Instruction

1. From a seated legs-apart position, bend the left knee in, supported, as in Head-to-Knee Pose (Janu Sirsasana). Keep the shoulders forward and let your right hand move down the inside of the right (straight) leg, but only go as far as you can without straining.

2. When you reach your limit, lift the left arm up towards the ceiling, keeping the shoulders moving on the angle of the straight leg, without turning the movement into a forward bend.

3. Hold for a few breaths.

4. Return in a controlled way, keeping the alignment.

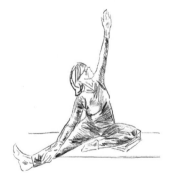

Teaching focus

- Correct posture.
- Side bend movement.
- Sitting into both 'sit' bones, not tipping over.
- Breathing into the stretch and opening up the ribcage.
- Allowing a sense of ease to come into the posture, while holding.

■ Revolved Side Angle Pose (Parivrtta Janu Sirsasana), with a strap

Instruction

1. Loop a strap around the foot of the straight leg, and bring it to the floor on the inside. As you slide your hand down the inside of your leg, catch hold of the strap as you stretch the other arm over.

■ Revolved Side Angle Pose (Parivrtta Janu Sirsasana), chair version

Instruction

1. On a chair with knees apart, turn a little to the left and aim the right shoulder at the right knee.

2. Take the right hand to the inside of the right knee, and slide it down the inside of the leg to the ankle.

3. Lift the left arm and continue to turn the body.

4. Hold for four breaths, and then repeat on the other side.

■ Half Spinal Twist Pose (Ardha Matsyendrasana) (seated twist)

This is a modification of the full practice familiar to all yoga teachers. Here we will explore easy stages, so that there is something that every individual can achieve, however immobile they may be.

This asana offers further opportunities to work the spine and to improve posture, to work the facet joints and to energise the whole structure. All of the twisting postures, whether seated or lying, act on the digestive organs by pressure and massage action throughout the abdomen. This improves peristalsis, enabling more efficient movement of food through the system (in yoga terms, improved Apana flow and therefore elimination). Manipura chakra is stimulated and energised. It is included here because of its action on the hips and pelvis connection, and the stretch it gives through the sciatic area.

Instruction

1. From the supported seated position on the floor, use blocks under the 'sit' bones and a block or blanket under the knees, as described in Staff Pose (Dandasana) (see page 60).

2. With the spine upright, turn the torso to each side alternately, simply placing both hands on the floor to the side. Do this slowly in your own time. (This will give the teacher time to observe and offer support.) Breathe with the movement, turning on the out-breath.

3. Then draw up the right knee, place the foot next to the left knee, hold on to the knee with both hands and draw the spine up and sit up.

4. Hold on to the knee with the left hand and extend the right hand forward at shoulder height; turn towards the knee, drawing it as close to the body as possible.

5. Sweep the right arm around to the back, placing that hand on the ground or on a block or perched on fingertips.

6. Let the head and neck join in the movement to look back over the shoulder. Use the eye muscles as well.

7. Hold and breathe in; encourage a little more turn on the out-breath. Return and repeat with the left knee bent and right leg straight.

8. Then cross the foot over the knee and repeat the twist with the same instruction, focus and guidance.

Some students may attempt the full posture, but it may require more hands-on help and care with the spinal posture. Note that the leg position of the full posture may be contraindicated for some types of hip replacement. Remember that the object of practice is not achievement of the full posture, but to practise enough to bring health benefits.

Teaching focus

- The spine should remain upright, and not slump back, even if this means a less strong turn.

- Encourage releasing and turning on the out-breath.

- Breathing up and down the spine, visualise the twisting action as an energy flowing up and down.

- Stay anchored in the tailbone and 'sit' bones.

- Encourage the placement of the abdomen against the leg, feeling the breath in the belly creating a massage action.

- Energising Manipura chakra.

LYING POSTURES FOR THE HIPS

The floor can be a great guide and support in many ways. In people with mobility challenges, just getting to the floor can be an effort. In the classroom, plan the order of postures to make maximum use of time on the floor and time and effort transferring, as for some this can be a workout in itself. Often a class might start on the floor using the floor-based warm-ups (see page 54).

◼ Floor Tree

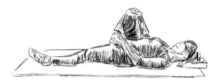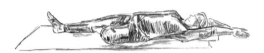

This posture is fun to try as an alternative to the standing balance 'tree' posture, Vrksasana. Obviously it does not provide the same balancing opportunity, but it does enable a different sense of alignment using the floor.

Instruction

1. Lie in a straight line, bend one knee up and place the foot next to the other leg, wherever it is comfortable.

2. Let the knee open out to the side – support the knee with blocks if the hip is stiff.

3. For those with more hip flexibility, the foot could be brought on to the top of the opposite groin, the folded knee moving out and down.

4. Do not over-arch the lower back or strain the knee. Arms can then be taken up above the head.

◼ Belly Twist Pose (Jathara Parivartanasana) (reclining twist)

This twisting action has long been known as a posture that frees up the lumbar area. It stretches the quadratus lumborum and psoas, and can help free up the lumbar vertebrae. It will support samana vayu and activate the energies of Manipura chakra at the level of Annamaya kosha. In both MS and Parkinson's students, the digestive process can be sluggish as the muscular action of digestion is impaired. The twisting action of this posture will provide a massage action on the gut to encourage movement.

There are stages in applying this asana, and we begin with the easiest, starting in semi-supine.

Instruction

1. Lying with the knees bent, and head supported, so that the neck has alignment, depending on the space available, stretch both arms out along the floor at shoulder level. If there is not room to do this, have the elbows bent, and hands cupping the back of the head.

2. Start the movement by taking the knees part of the way to the left, on an exhale breath – moving to the left first exerts a little pressure on the rising colon, and works the body in a way that optimises the passage of food through the digestive tract.

3. Bring the knees back to the centre on an inhale breath.

4. Move the knees over to the right, exhaling.

5. This can be repeated two or three times, gradually increasing the twisting action until the legs are going as far over as is possible within a pain-free range. The shoulders should stay on the floor so that the upper body is stable. Head turning can be added to complete the twist action, but only if the student is comfortable with this.

6. Once the posture becomes familiar, move into a longer hold, with gentle normal breathing, allowing time for release in the joints and muscles.

7. Come out of the posture when you are ready (this encourages awareness).

The following variations may offer slightly different actions:

1. Offer a block to be held between the knees, and encourage squeezing it on the turn, focusing on the adductors, and encourage engagement of the pelvic floor.

2. A harder option is to slide the left leg straight and take the right leg over and across the body. This may require a pile of blocks to support the knee and take the strain.

3. This also offers an opportunity for a hand-on easing, if the student is comfortable with that. Place a hand on the shoulder, but do not force – just aid the student in keeping it in place. The other hand can help the hip, giving a diagonal stretch. Do this incrementally, with the student's permission. Many students find that with hands on to guide, release can happen more easily.

Teaching focus

- Alignment of the spine, head and neck – the shoulders stay on the floor.
- A massage action on the digestive tract.
- Visualise spinal release.
- Visualise the space between the hip bone and armpit, and breathe into the space.
- Explain the action of samana vayu.
- While the posture is held, visualise the muscle lengthening and softness spreading through tight areas. Visualise samana vayu as warmth spreading around the stomach area.

Parkinson's note: It may be difficult for some to move very far because of rigidity in the spine. Support may be needed with a folded blanket under the back.

WORKING THE HIPS IN STANDING POSTURES

Providing the student is able to stand, working the hip joint in an upright position gives an opportunity for balancing as well as hip mobilising.

Place a chair on the mat for support, so that the back of the chair can be easily reached.

◼ Semi-squat

This will begin to bring awareness into the hip movement and also strengthen the thighs.

Instruction

1. Stand facing the chair back, about an arm's length away. You can hold it if need be.

2. Keeping your feet and knees parallel, feel where your hip joint is – you will bend from here.

3. Draw up the pelvic floor and engage the abdominal muscles.

4. Send the tailbone back as you bend, and bring your arms forward to touch the chair back, or have them stretched out in front of you.

5. Return to upright and repeat four times

Teaching focus

- Strength and core engagement.

- Keeping parallel alignment.

- Confidence in sitting.

◼ Step over walk

Instruction

1. Stand with the feet parallel and with the chair to the left, and lightly hold the back of the chair with your left hand.

2. Establish the standing leg and foot, to be strong and firm.

3. Lift the right leg with the knee bent out to the side, and then lift higher up and forward, as if you are stepping over a low obstacle.

4. Repeat this movement four times, and then circle the hip as if you are stepping backwards. Lift the leg up around and back. Repeat four times in this direction.

Do this with the other leg.

Teaching focus

- Encourage a high lift to the leg.

- Good rooting into the ground through the standing foot and leg.

- Focus on the movement of the hip.

- Be aware of the upper body and observe if there is compensating action through the spine and body movement in order to accomplish the action. Encourage steadiness.

- Balance and confidence.

LUNGING

Lunges both flex and extend the hip and stretch the psoas and iliopsoas, which is necessary to keep the hips mobile. There are often issues with balance and stability for those with MS and Parkinson's, which will rule out the full standing postures. Working supported versions will help those students who are less able.

▓ Lunging posture from Cat Pose

Instruction

1. Place a blanket under the knees for padding.

2. Bring your right foot forward.

3. Place your hands either side of the foot.

4. Rock backwards and forwards, gradually working into a deeper lunge.

5. As you become stronger, hands can be placed on the hips; this then becomes a more challenging posture as balance is involved.

6. Gradually try to hold the posture in the lunge position. One this is mastered, your arms can be brought into Namaste or even raised.

All the variations and advances can be offered as choices, so that each student can work to their own ability.

▓ Lunging postures using a chair for support

Many lunging postures such as Extended Side Angle Pose (Utthita Parsvakonasana) can be modified using a chair. The chair method offers stability and a means of allowing the opportunity to try complex movements requiring coordination, balance and mobility that may not always be achievable in unsupported versions.

There are stages that can be offered so that students can feel their way. This helps to build confidence.

■ Hip easing for lunges

Instruction

1. Place the chair on the mat, with the seat facing to the right, side on, so that you can place your foot on the seat, in the middle, and hold the back of the chair. Check that the chair will not tip if you press your weight into it.

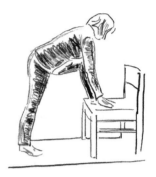

2. Keep the back leg straight if possible, with the heel pressing firmly on the floor, and rock in towards the chair. This gives a deep knee bend in the right knee and a stretch in the left hamstring.

3. Move back and forth with a gentle rock, easing out the joints. Then change to the other leg.

4. To deepen the stretch, move a little further away from the chair, to stretch further.

5. When you gain confidence, try placing both hands on the bent knee. Hold the chair to keep steady if needed.

6. Lift one hand up, and then, if the balance can be held, lift the other. Bring the arms back down.

7. Keep steady with the help of the chair to bring your foot back to the floor.

8. Repeat on the other leg.

9. Counter-pose with a Seated Forward Bend (Paschimottanasana).

Teaching focus

- Allow the students to find their own level.

- Hip action and lengthening through the hamstrings.

- Encourage grounding, focus, balance and stability.

- Keep the upper body lifted and chest open.

Parkinson's note: People with Parkinson's can often droop forward over the chair and lean in, so encourage upright upper body, and keep the movement in the hips.

Yoga practice that brings awareness of the spine establishes core stability. Keeping the framework of the shoulder girdle and pelvis open and mobile will build a foundation for some of the superstretches, balancing and flow sequences that add to the variety of practices that can be offered and begin to bring enjoyment in practice.

Balancing

The ability to balance depends on the ears, eyes and proprioception. Fluids in the semicircular canals of the inner ears shift with our body movements and, through the sensitivity of fine hairs in the semicircular canals, send messages to the brain about the positioning of the head. Vision helps us to orientate to external reference points. Proprioception relies on information from sensory receptors in the joints and muscles in the body, and via skin pressure to ascertain the position of the body, and enables adjustment to be made. In people with MS and Parkinson's, this messaging system is impaired. This means that balance becomes a major issue; falls and their consequences – broken bones, bruising and then the stress on the body of repairing – is a major health concern.

As well as loss of control over the proprioception messaging system, there is loss of coordination and confusion in the nerve messaging system, ordering the body to act in set sequences; this results in loss of confidence and strength. Students become fearful of losing balance, of stumbling and falling, and give up trying to perform the things that would be helpful. Some of the medications given such as muscle relaxants, sedatives and blood pressure drugs can cause dizziness and light-headedness, and a combination of these makes things worse.

Therapeutic yoga builds strength and confidence, and puts in place safe support to enable students to overcome their fear. Many with MS will be unable to stand or balance without support, but, with support, transferring and bearing weight with practice will strengthen the body. It is essential that balance practices are given regularly and that students build week by week to ensure progress. Their muscles will become stronger, and they will get better at knowing when they are off balance.

In general, students should be encouraged to take long strides, and to keep the shoulders over the hips and to stand tall.

Overall, balancing practices can brings improvement in the following ways:

- becoming calmer
- stretches the shoulders and neck
- tones the legs and buttocks
- improves digestion
- reduces fatigue and alleviates insomnia
- strengthens the thighs, calves, ankles and spine
- stretches the groins and inner thighs, chest and shoulders
- improves the sense of balance
- relieves sciatica and reduces flat feet
- improves concentration

- strengthens wrists, arms and shoulders

- improves upper body and core strength

- creates good posture.

FEELING THE WAY

■ Balance and off-balance

Instruction

1. Stand in Mountain Pose (Tadasana) (see page 78), and encourage awareness and focus.

2. Bring a chair to the side, and check that it will not slide away and that the back of the chair is at a handy height to hold if needed, or place the chair in front so that it can be held with both hands. Alternatively, stand by a wall.

3. Taking awareness into the feet, sense how the weight of the body is carried into both feet. Notice any differences between left and right, and encourage an even spread between both.

4. Connect with the floor through the outside edges of each foot, and around into the little toe.

■ Transferring weight, side to side and backwards and forwards

This helps build awareness and confidence.

Instruction

1. Slowly lean a little to the right, taking the weight on to the right foot, until you feel you might fall, then pull yourself back into balance. This way you can train the muscles and nerve perception to bring yourself back upright.

2. Do the same on the other side.

3. Try the same exploration, but backwards and forwards this time. Lean forwards slightly, towards the toes and then pulling back – feel for the place on the edge of falling.

4. Lean back a little and then pull back to full balance. Start with small movements. You are training proprioception.

Teaching focus

- Let the students continue to repeat the actions, and encourage them to explore their own limits of staying in balance and to feel for how they correct themselves to return to balance.

■ Back and forth

Another way of building confidence in balance is to encourage transferring weight from one foot to the other, backwards and forwards, using an 'easy step' forward (see page 80). With a chair alongside, let the student step on to the front leg, shifting their weight forward, and then rocking on to the back foot.

MINI BALANCES

Holding a wall or chair initially provides a sense of security and support. As the weeks go by, we can encourage a lighter touch on the support, allowing the strength in the body to take the responsibility for being upright.

Instruction

1. Take time to prepare and focus. Use the idea of growing roots and feeling that the supporting leg is strong and sturdy. If we can engage the mind and intention in a positive way, our progress is enhanced.

2. Bend and lift one knee, lifting the other foot off the floor. Place it back down with full mindfulness in the action of placing the foot back onto the ground. Do the same on the other leg.

3. Hold the leg up for a little longer.

4. Extend the leg and hold it a little off the floor.

5. Add point and flex foot action. This will extend the holding time, as well as working the muscles of the lower leg and foot.

6. Progress to extending the heel, circling the whole leg from the hip.

All of these additional movements build up strength and confidence. Aim to keep the body steady throughout.

Teaching focus

- Remind the students to breathe (people forget when they are concentrating hard).

- Keep the focus in the feet.

- Encourage the gaze to be forwards rather than down.

- Let the upper body stay relaxed.

- Establish confidence by progressing to more challenging and longer balancing practices before attempting the modified versions of the classical yoga balances.

■ Back leg lift

Instruction

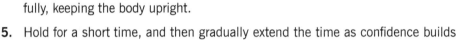

1. The chair should be placed with the back alongside, within easy reach.

2. Hold the chair with one hand and place the other hand on the hip, and take an 'easy step' forward (see page 80).

3. Continue to transfer the weight forward on a bent knee, so that the back foot slowly lifts off the floor.

4. Move through easy stages, first with the tip of the toe on the floor, and then allow the foot to lift fully, keeping the body upright.

5. Hold for a short time, and then gradually extend the time as confidence builds and leg strength improves.

6. To come out of the pose, place the toe on the floor and gently rock the weight back until the whole of the back foot is on the floor, spreading the weight throughout both legs and feet.

7. Repeat on the other side.

8. In time you can progress to standing without the chair. Place your hands on your hips, shifting your weight forwards and gradually taking your back foot off the ground. Keep the chair in place for safety.

Teaching focus

- Grounding: the front foot will take the weight so make sure it is firmly planted, toes spreading.

- The knees should remain aligned in the direction of the mid toe and ankle; do not allow the knees to roll in.

- The knees can stay bent.

- Encourage long smooth breathing.

Parkinson's note: Breaking down the movement into step-by-step actions helps the brain to order the messaging to the body.

■ Front leg lift

Instruction

1. With the chair to support, lift one bent knee up. Hold for a short time (this can be adjusted according to need). Repeat on the other side.

2. Repeat and open the bent knee out to the side. Repeat on the other side.

3. Extend the balance by having one hand on the back of the chair to keep steady and lift a knee up in front. Hold it with the free hand.

4. Draw this knee up and in towards the body as close as possible, giving a deep flexion in the knee joint.

5. Hold for just a short time before repeating on the other leg.

◼ Lord of the Dance Pose (Natarajasana)

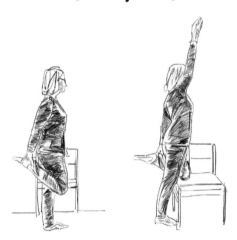

Instruction
Preliminary Stork Pose:

1. Place a chair to the side for support, or stand next to a wall.

2. Think of the standing leg and foot, and feel that they are strong and firm.

3. Breathe out and contract the abdominal muscles, and draw up the pelvic floor, creating a strong core in the balance.

4. Bend one knee up in front and hold it with your hand, slide the hand towards the ankle and move the knee down and back, bringing the leg in as close as possible, heel to buttocks.

5. Keep the gaze steady, focusing on a point in front of you.

6. Keeping the spine long and hips level, draw the knee back as far as possible while keeping your balance.

7. Come out of the pose, step by step. Let go of the leg, place the foot on the floor, and spread the weight evenly over both feet.

8. As you find stability, you can experiment with letting go of the chair or wall. From the Stork Pose you can progress to an adapted form of Dancer Pose. It is safer to use the wall for support. Ability to do this posture will depend on whether the ankle can be held.

9. To return from the pose, lower the arm if it is lifted, lift the spine upright and lower the leg back to the floor. Make a good connection through the feet before letting go of any support.

■ Modified Dancer Pose

Instruction

1. Stand facing the wall; a chair may be too low to do this safely. Have enough space in front to accommodate a bend forward, or stand alongside the wall so that one hand can hold it throughout.

2. Take up the Stork Pose (see above).

3. Tilt forward and place the free hand on the wall. This will be enough of a challenge at first. This movement will give an opportunity to check the alignment of the hips, pelvis and spine.

4. Focus your gaze either at the fingertips or a point on the wall ahead.

Teaching focus

- Feel a strength through the feet, and keep them well rooted.

- Keep the gaze steady, looking at a still point.

- Don't tip sideways in the hips or over-arch the back.

- Engage the core.

- The chest should be up and forward.

- Feel light.

- Go step by step and give permission to stop at any stage.

- If the ankle cannot be held behind, it may be possible for the student to catch hold of the bottom of their yoga pants/trousers. Do not use a strap, because if the student loses balance, they could easily fall by being caught up in the strap.

- Allow students to find their own way at first, to build confidence, and give teaching points to encourage correct alignment. Being able to do this in any form is a real achievement for people with limited movement.

- You can gradually develop this over the weeks, encouraging the back bend element of the posture, its grace and steadiness. Give lots of encouragement and keep comments light-hearted.

Parkinson's/MS note: Hands-on help for aligning and positioning the hips and shoulders is of great help in balancing postures. It serves as another point of reference in the bio feedback of the senses.

■ Dancer Pose, chair-supported version

This gives attention to the back-bending aspect of the balance, and the length and openness through the front of the body from the knee up to the shoulders, but without the difficulty of the leg-back action.

Instruction

1. Place a chair with the back at the right-hand side for support. Place a block or cushion on the chair seat to get it at the right height.

2. Hold the back of the chair with the right hand and place the right knee on the seat/block.

3. Extend the left arm up and move the hips forward, creating a mild back arch. Breathe in and stretch up.

4. Look up, moving the head slowly.

5. Lower the arm, and repeat the stretching action three times. Relax and bring your knee off the seat.

6. Repeat with the left knee on the seat (moving to the other side of the chair is the easiest way).

7. Progress the stretch by lifting the heel of the standing foot to be on your toes as you stretch up.

Teaching focus

- Keep the gaze ahead.

- Make sure that the chair is at the right height.

- Hold the student steady at the hips if they are feeling wobbly.

- Give permission to come out of the pose at any time or to opt out completely if they do not feel stable enough to try it.

■ Tree Pose (Vrksasana)

This is an excellent posture for developing a sense of balance and strength. It can be offered in steps so that there is something that everyone can do, which fosters a sense of achievement and confidence.

Preliminary tree balance:

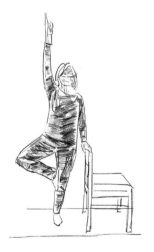

Instruction

1. Use a chair or the wall for support.

2. Stand with your feet together. Turn one foot out slightly and lift the heel to place over the instep of the other foot.

3. While holding the chair for safety and steadiness, lengthen your spine, and grow imaginary roots down through the feet into the ground.

4. Take time to stand unaided if possible, bringing the palms together in front of the chest to complete the pose.

When sufficient confidence is gained, move on to practise without a chair.

Instruction

1. With the same safety measures in place as before, lift one leg until the foot touches a little way up the side of the leg.

2. Find the placement that feels right for you. There should be no straining.

3. Turn the knee out, but only within the range that is comfortable for hip mobility.

4. Aid stamina in the pose by engaging your core muscles and using breathing.

5. Hold for a number of breaths – start with three and gradually build up. This can give you a measure of improvement over the weeks, as you are able to hold for a greater number of breaths.

6. You can then choose whether to work unaided.

7. The arms can be used in different positions; if support is still in use, the other arm can be lifted above the head, out to shoulder height, or held on or in front of the chest.

8. The gaze should be held steady on a point straight ahead, to aid concentration (drishti). I prefer to use a point on the wall or another place on a level with the gaze rather than on, say, the fingertips.

9. Check the position of the head and neck, keeping the neck long and the chin level.

10. Return from the posture in a controlled manner. Bring the spine upright, lower the arms and leg, in a smooth movement. Plant both feet back on the floor.

11. Counter-pose by releasing the spine in a soft forward bend.

Teaching focus

- Long spine, growing tall.
- Engage the core muscles, strong trunk.
- Alignment: the pelvis should be level; check the spine in case of over-arching or a contracting lumbar spine.
- Ground through the feet – visualise roots.
- Strong legs, but don't jam the knees.
- Steady breathing throughout.
- Soft shoulders and shoulder blades moving down the back.

▮ Tree Pose with chair support

Other options within this posture could be to offer an opportunity to work with the upper body, with both arms lifted, and to lift the leg higher by using a chair to support the foot. In this adaptation a chair is placed with the seat side on to the student.

Instruction

1. Place one foot on the chair seat; this gives security and a different feel to the balance. Some people may still need to hold the wall or the back of the chair to start with.

2. Lift the spine upright and bring in the arm positions.

3. With a foot securely on the chair, the arm action can be directed in several different ways – palms together, arms stretching upwards, or with parallel arms extended upwards or out at shoulder height.

4. Hold steady in the pose, for several breaths.

5. Adjust any arm positions to accommodate any shoulder issues.

Teaching focus

- Breath.
- Grounding and stability.
- Strength.
- Concentration.

■ Side arm and leg lift

Instruction

1. Hold a chair or wall for support. Lift one leg out to the side and at the same time lift the arm on the same side.

2. Keep the body still, hips and shoulders in parallel while carrying out the arm/ leg movements.

Teaching focus

- Although the balancing postures are often a challenge, it is important to make the practice enjoyable. Make light of wobbles and 'strange shapes' – each individual is making their own unique posture.

■ Warrior Pose balance

There are various ways to offer this posture with a chair for support.

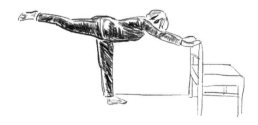

Instruction

1. Stand facing the back of the chair, and with both hands on the chair take a step back.

2. Engage the core.

3. Lift one leg back and up, leaning towards the chair, and stay steady, using the hands.

4. When you become comfortable with the pose, try a deeper forward bend and higher leg lift. Extend the practice by reaching one arm forward over the back of the chair.

5. Once you gain confidence, turn the chair around with the seat facing, put both hands on the seat and lift one leg up and back, progressing to lifting one arm, and then both.

6. To return, lower the leg, bend the knees and shift the weight back to establish balance on both feet, before lifting the spine and letting go of the chair.

7. Repeat on the other foot.

Teaching focus

- Maintain focus, steady gaze and steady breathing.

- Put roots down through the supporting foot and have confidence in the strength of the supporting leg and foot.

- Engage core muscles.

- Go only as far as the student is confident.

- Encourage grounding and putting roots down from the feet into the ground. Stimulate Apana vayu.

- Watch out for tipping hips and correct this gently.

- Engage the pelvic floor and strengthen the glutes for a good lift.

■ Floor balances

Balances can be offered from the floor as well as in a standing position. These offer a different way of building strength, and still depend on a strong sense of grounding and a strong centre.

Make sure that students are sitting away from the wall, in case they roll back.

Instruction

1. Sit on the floor (not on a block), with knees bent and your hands holding under and behind your knees.

2. Very gradually, lean back and feel for the place of balance; lift your heels so that you are on tiptoes, and then lift the feet so that you are balanced.

3. Hold there for a few moments to get the feel of being able to hold the balance.

4. Experiment with whether you are able to lift one foot higher, keeping the knee bent, and then try the other leg.

5. Progress to lifting both heels together, and then taking the hands away.

6. If you are stronger, you will be able to move on to attempting to straighten the legs.

7. Return by simply placing your feet back on the floor.

◼ Chair balance

Instruction

1. Sit upright on your 'sit' bones, and hold the seat with your hands.

2. Engage the core muscles.

3. Press your heels into the floor as if you are trying to pick your toes up.

4. Hold your lower leg in that position, while trying to maintain parallel knees, and lift your feet off the floor, one at a time. Then try lifting both together.

5. Progress to extending your arms out to the sides and holding for a few breaths.

6. Try different hand positions – for example, palms together and lifting them up, or raising arms in parallel.

Teaching focus

*   Focus strongly in Muladhara.
*   Engage the core.
*   Build confidence and stamina.

◼ Cat Pose balance

Instruction

1. From the standard Cat Pose (see page 51), take your weight evenly over all four contact points.

2. Inhale and exhale, drawing in the abdominals, and engage the pelvic floor.

3. Lift the right hand about 5 cm (3 inches) off the floor, and at the same time bring the left knee forward and lift about 5 cm (3 inches).

4. Hold stable on the two diagonals of opposing hand and foot.

5. Try to keep your hips level and hold the pose. Keep the muscles active and breathe normally.

6. Place the hand and knee down, and then repeat on the other side.

7. Do this a few times over, according to your own stamina.

Teaching focus

- Core strength.
- Steadiness and breathing.
- Check that hips are level.
- Long spine, long neck.

Superstretches

One of the most popular benefits of yoga practice, reported by all of those with Parkinson's and MS that I have ever worked with, is the good feeling that is induced by stretching. When muscles are in spasm and there is great rigidity, stretching can bring immense relief and release. Working with symmetry will help those who have become lopsided, even though some of the asanas are complicated; 'having a go' promotes a positive feeling.

The stretches on pages 40–55 should be used as a warm-up.

SIDE BENDING AND TRIANGLE POSE (TRIKONASANA)

Many yoga teachers are familiar with this stretch that lengthens the obliques, latissimus dorsi, quadratus lumborum and opens up the intercostal muscles. In this position we can encourage breathing coordination. These improve the lateral bend of the spine, open the intercostals and promote elasticity in respiration.

The Triangle Pose and extended Triangle Pose give a superb stretch throughout the whole body, centring on the heart with the limbs radiating out. A strong grounded posture and open-hearted energy flow can be established.

■ Easy side bend

Often used as a warm-up before Triangle Pose, this easy side bend is useful in its own right and enables the student to explore their range of side bending in the spine, gently beginning to stretch the inner thighs.

Instruction

1. Stand with the back of a chair facing you, feet apart, a little wider than the hips, arms down by the sides.

2. Slide one hand down the leg, just as far as you can go, while keeping the spine as if you are standing with your back against the wall. If there is wall space in the room, try practising the posture against the wall. This will provide extra support and keep good alignment.

3. Return to an upright position and repeat on the other side.

4. Do this five times, slowly.

Teaching focus

- Bring awareness to any differences between right and left, and support the students in working in a balanced way.

- Bring awareness into where the body is moving and stretching.

- This posture can be done standing with the back against the wall, if balance is an issue.

■ Progressing the posture

There are various ways to progress in this posture.

Instruction

1. Increase the stretch by lifting an arm up and lengthening away to the sky, and from that long place move the spine laterally, keeping the feet and legs steady without losing grounding.

2. Repeat the movements in the first instance, and then try holding for a number of breaths – three or four is often enough to build stability. Release early from the pose if needed.

3. The stretch can be extended a little more by widening the stride. Holding the back of the chair with one hand can help the shoulders and chest to stay facing forward. Place the right hand in the centre of the chair back and lift the left hand while bending to the right. This helps to keep the lower shoulder down and forward as the other reaches up and over; alignment is then maintained.

Variations can be offered to help with spine and shoulder awareness. If there is a frozen shoulder issue or immobility for some other reason, a hand can be placed on the hip, as the spine moves into the bend.

Teaching focus

- In wide-leg postures it is important to engage the core muscles, to promote inner strength and good posture.

- Make sure the spine is not twisting forward or back.

- Breathe into the ribs.

- This posture gives the teacher an opportunity to guide gently with a hand on the shoulder using words to encourage, rather than pulling or pushing. Light touch and gentle instruction are enough to bring attention to the posture and encourage stretching and opening.

- We can remind the body how it needs to adjust, even if we repeat the same instructions week by week. Thus we can check:

  - the mobility of the spine

  - that the hips and pelvis are not twisting

  - the position and alignment of the head and shoulders

  - that extra attention is given to where there is rigidity, muscle spasm and immobility.

■ Supported Triangle Pose

This version with chair support offers greater stability and a secure base from which to stretch.

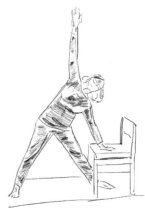

Instruction

1. Using a chair for support, place the chair on the mat, seat facing you.

2. Stand facing the chair and place the right foot on the floor under the chair seat. Step as wide as you can while still feeling steady. Work within your own limitations and hip mobility.

3. According to your balance and steadiness, the next step is to lift the arms to shoulder height. Allow the front knee to bend if it is tight – do not strain to make it straight.

4. Lengthen out to the side through the waist, and place the right hand on the seat of the chair.

5. To lift out gracefully, extend the arm and bring the spine upright.

6. Repeat on the other side.

Teaching focus

- Encourage alignment and guide actions by offering instruction in words, before starting to make any hands-on adjustments.

- Check the alignment of the head and neck, keeping the neck long, and avoid jutting the chin out.

- Check that the posture is a side bend, with no forward twisting.

- Offer modification to rest the upward arm, elbow bent, hand on hip. This is especially useful if there has been a shoulder injury.

- Encourage the chest to be open and the breath to fill the chest.

- Anahata awareness.

Parkinson's/MS note: Many people with Parkinson's have problems with rigidity of the neck, so take special care with head movements as they can sometimes affect balance and cause dizziness. Students with sufficient balance and steadiness can work a standard Triangle Pose without the chair.

FORWARD BENDS

■ Work at the wall, half forward bend

If there is sufficient wall space, get the students to stand facing the wall. A chair may suffice for shorter people.

Instruction

1. Reach forward to put both hands on the wall, step back, and have your feet a little wider than your hips. Lengthen your tailbone back and extend your upper back.

2. Come out of the posture in your own time. To come out, simply step towards the wall.

3. Counter-pose with a gentle twist from a standing, sitting or lying position to release the spine.

Teaching focus

• Let your student know what you are seeing. Giving positive feedback even for the tiniest achievements creates a 'feel good' factor and builds confidence.

• Move the posture along by encouraging a deeper stretch and giving breathing instructions.

• Bring students into inner awareness to feel into the stretch release options.

Contraindication: This posture is hugely beneficial for the spine and a great stretch for the hamstrings, but caution is needed if the spine has kyphosis or severe scoliosis or if there are shoulder injuries.

Parkinson's note: Students with Parkinson's are often in a state of spasm in the upper back, and they commonly have kyphosis, created mostly from muscle rigidity, rather than bone misalignment. Work gently with the idea of lengthening, moving the shoulder blades down the back, aiming to create a 'hollow' in the thoracic spine. A hand placed lightly on the area where you are encouraging movement will help focus. If a wall is not available, this stretch can be done with the support of a chair back, but its effectiveness of ease and alignment will be related to the height of the student.

■ Further hamstring stretches

Instruction

1. Standing about 30 cm (1 foot) away from the wall, engage the abdominal muscles and the pelvic floor, keeping the body as straight as possible.

2. With arms forward and hands on the wall, bend the elbows and lean into the wall.

Teaching focus

- Look for the body sagging, and encourage work into the abdominals; check the shoulder position.

- Check that the heels are down – a wedge-shaped block might help here if there is strong shortening of the Achilles tendon.

- Ask the student to stand near to the wall and to put their hands and forearms on the wall at shoulder height, elbows bent. They should walk the hand upwards bit by bit, keeping the shoulder blades down and the body straight and flat.

■ Rag Doll Pose (forward bend)

This is an easy roll-down bend, and there are many versions that will be familiar to yoga teachers.

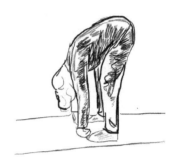

Instruction

Version 1:

1. Reach your arms up and extend the spine, lifting up out of the hips. Soften everything and melt down, bending your knees as you go.

Version 2:

1. Start with the chin in, and focus on curling the spine down, knees bending, and then hang loosely forward.

Contraindication: Some back problems, spinal pain, osteoporosis, sinusitis, headaches, high blood pressure, glaucoma or detached retina.

Teaching focus

- These movements allow the spine to open and create full flexion. Guide the student into slowly uncurling with awareness of the action of the spine.

- Letting go.

- Allow gravity to take over and experience a gentle downwards pull.

- Imagine the spine lengthening in a passive way.

- Keep the knees released.

- Grounding.

- Imagine the muscles lengthening.

- Offer alternatives to the above if a full bend is not possible or if there is instability. Place a chair in front of the student and encourage a gentle bend to put hands on the chair. If using a chair, with their hands on the knees, ask the student to bend forward within their capability, without straining, letting the body fold further, sliding their hands down to the feet.

Parkinson's note: It may be possible to stand behind a wobbly student and to hold their waist or hips (with permission), or even to use a strap around the hips to keep them steady while they experiment with bending. In class, this will be dependent on whether you have an assistant present. Any forward bending is useful in relieving rigidity in the spine.

MS note: If you are working with a student in a wheelchair, experiment with using a strap connected to the chair.

■ Standing Rag Doll Pose

After preparation with hamstring stretches, wall work or Rag Doll Pose, most students can achieve some level of active forward bending. For those who do not balance well or who have limitations such as back problems or high blood pressure, glaucoma or sinusitis, a chair can be placed in front of the student, or a sitting modification offered.

Instruction

1. Standing tall, begin by lengthening the spine and aligning in parallel through the feet, knees, hips and shoulders.

2. Inhale and raise the arms upwards, with a feeling of lifting up out of the hips.

3. Exhale as you bend forward from the hip joint, allowing the knees to bend if they are tight, letting the arms or elbows come to rest on the chair seat if the spine needs some support.

4. Lift out by walking the hands up the legs, to come upright.

Teaching focus

- Students can hold the position while it is comfortable and move deeper into the posture. Encourage a sense of releasing and letting go.

- This posture helps to ease out rigidity and spasm in the spine and lower back.

- Swadhistana and Muladhara chakras. Visualise these centres being activated; use a colour visualisation – orange or red, for example.

- Strengthens Apana vayu.

- Caution is needed for back injuries, prolapsed discs, sinusitis, glaucoma, detached retina and high blood pressure in the standard version.

FORWARD BEND VARIATIONS

◼ Adapted Wide-legged Forward Bend (Prasarita Padottanasana) (feet apart)

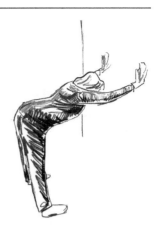

Having the feet apart gives another dimension to the stretch.

Instruction

1. Stand with the feet wide.

2. Bend forward from the hips and place your hands on your knees, further down your legs or ankles.

3. If your knees bend or roll inwards, adjust the width of the feet. Use a chair in front if this provides better stability.

Teaching focus

- Check for tight hamstrings, adductors and hips, and adjust the stride accordingly.

- Encourage the spine to lengthen.

- Visualise long supple muscles, stretching with ease.

◼ Intense Side Stretch Pose (Parsvottanasana) (One-Leg Forward Bend)

Yoga teachers will be aware of this classic – it is good grounding and a great hamstring stretch, promoting strength in the legs and building confidence.

Here is an adapted version using a chair for support, although this may not be needed in all cases. Using a chair enables the student with Parkinson's or MS to work safely and begin to stretch, supporting the spine.

Instruction

1. Place the chair on the mat in front of you.

2. Begin with parallel feet and take an 'easy step' forward (see page 80), placing the forward foot just under the chair. Turn the back foot out slightly to the side.

3. Take your hands to the hip joint (teachers can demonstrate where this is). This is where the body will begin to bend.

4. Let the spine begin to lengthen, and keep lengthening as you inhale.

5. As you exhale, bend forwards at the hip.

6. Let the hands move slowly down the leg, bit by bit. This can act as support, but direct the asana so that there is no pressure through the hands, and so that the spine is active.

7. Let the bend continue so that the legs begin to stretch; when the knee wants to bend, let it.

8. Your hands can come to rest on the seat of the chair while you hold the stretch a little longer.

9. Come up slowly, walking the hands up the leg if the back is weak. Lifting out of this posture also offers a chance to continue working with the spine and breath.

10. Repeat a couple of times, and then change sides.

Teaching focus

- Students should work within their own limits – it is important not to strain. Use Ahimsa.

- Grounding and balance.

- Explore the stretch and breathe into it.

- Visualise elasticity.

- Swadhistana and Muladhara chakras.

- Apana vayu.

- Offer a mild back bend as a counter-pose, such as arms held behind the back and chest lifted, neck supported, by gently tucking the chin in. This can be offered in a sitting position if needed.

■ Intense Side Stretch Pose (Parsvottanasana), seated version

Instruction

1. Sit towards the front of the chair, making sure you are sitting up on the 'sit' bones. Stretch one leg out – this can be supported by putting your heel on a block (two blocks will make it harder).

2. Place your hands first on the hip joint, to become aware that this is where the movement will start.

3. Inhale. Exhale as you lean forward from the hip joint, lengthening the spine.

4. Take both hands onto the thigh of the straight leg, keeping the spine long and straight.

5. Slide your hands down towards the knee, and further if possible. Let the spine stay long and keep the stretch in the hamstrings, letting the knee bend if it wants to.

6. Go as far as possible and hold a little at the end of the stretch, with steady breathing.

7. Return to upright and repeat on the other leg.

If more stretch is needed, stand facing a chair. Place your foot on the chair seat with your leg straight.

1. Stand tall and breathe in, exhale and lengthen the spine as you bend forward over the straight leg; slide your hand down toward the knee, going as far as you can.

2. Hold the stretch, visualising the muscles releasing and lengthening.

3. Repeat on the other side.

■ One-arm extended fold

Instruction

1. With the seat of a chair facing you, place one foot forward under the chair.

2. Place one hand behind your back and extend the other upwards.

3. Bend forward from the hips, paying attention to the shoulder and spine position.

4. The extended arm can rest on the chair back; with this support, more awareness can be brought into the spine.

5. Return to the starting position, or bring both hands to the chair as you come upright.

6. Repeat four times.

7. Practise on the other side.

Teaching focus

- This posture can help where there is scoliosis of the spine – both sides should be worked equally.

- Bring awareness to any one-sidedness that is often a symptom of Parkinson's, and correct the alignment.

WARMS-UPS FOR SEATED FORWARD BEND (PASCHIMOTTANASANA)

■ Back and forth and rowing

Props are helpful in this posture. Sit on a block if the hip joints and lower back are tight, and use a rolled blanket to support under the knees if the hamstrings are tight and the legs cannot be comfortably straight.

Instruction

1. Lift your arms forwards, to shoulder height, parallel with the floor.

2. Exhale and engage the core muscles.

3. Inhale and lean back a little way, and then ease forward, while lengthening the spine and breathing out. Reach the arms forward and then pull back, breathing in. A block could be held to give steadiness.

4. This can be extended into a 'rowing' action. Draw the arms in, elbows out, as you lean back, as if pulling on oars, and then stretch the arms up and over on the forward bend.

■ Seated Forward Bend (Paschimottanasana)

First check if there are any spinal problems that may be contraindicated, such as acute prolapsed disc, degeneration in the spine or osteoporosis. Offer a block to sit on and support under the knees.

Instruction

1. Start as in the preliminary stretch (see previous exercise) engage the core, ease the back, and raise the arms above your head. Lift up out of the pelvis and lengthen the spine – imagine reaching for a trapeze bar just above your head.

2. As you exhale, move from the hips, bending forward over the legs. Let your arms come to rest somewhere on the legs or feet. Actively move your shoulder blades down into the back ribs.

3. Come out of the pose by releasing softly over the legs, letting the arms trail along the floor, building the spine up.

4. For a counter-pose, do a simple back bend.

Teaching focus

- Don't let the students struggle with the goal of catching hold of their toes or trying to put their head on their knees. When a bend that is within their own range is attained, encourage breathing and lengthening.

- Breathe into the stretch along the back of the body.

- Imagine the spine lengthening – direct the crown of the head towards the toes.

- Check the spine is not over-arched or the neck compressed.

- Imagine a line down the front of the body, and keep it long.

- Let the shoulders relax and soften.

- Allow the knees to bend.

- Breathe light into Swadisthana chakra.

Parkinson's/MS note: It is helpful to be hands-on. Encourage an upright spine to allow the student to feel the difference and to 'know' their own capabilities, identifying what needs to change and how to action that change. Placing a hand lightly on part of the back to encourage length and lift will give guidance and enable the student to respond. The ability to 'do' the posture is almost irrelevant, as it is the enquiry into the body that will start to bring the biggest benefits.

Give encouragement, however small the improvement might be. In any arm-lifting movement that occurs frequently in many postures, it is important to take into account the shape of the spine and any shoulder injuries or frozen shoulder conditions. In an effort to extend arms above, students will often facilitate this action by over-arching the spine and neck, creating a false feeling of lift, when what is actually happening is a distortion; this is harmful if repeated often, and can cause strain in the spine and in the shoulders. Make sure that the movement is actioned from the correct joint and the shoulder extension is not forced but kept within the student's mobility range.

It may be possible to give a little assistance by standing and holding the student's hands in an up and forward direction, checking as you go that it is not too much. Ask the student to tell you when to stop, but be sensitive for resistance through the arms and shoulders that will tell you how far to go.

■ Wide-Angle Seated Forward Bend (Upavista Konasana) (legs-apart stretch sequence)

Rather than using this as a static posture, I suggest a set of bends that enable the muscles to stretch gently within the movement.

Instruction

1. Sit up on the block, with your legs apart, and feel into the 'sit' bones; your legs can remain bent.

2. Within your own limits, turn your body to the right leg.

3. Inhale, lean back a little, stretch your arms up and then exhale, bending from the hips to fold over the right leg, as far as is possible, without straining.

4. Release almost immediately and return to the sitting-up position.

5. Repeat on the left side. Facing front, breathe in, lean back, stretch the arms up and lift the ribcage.

6. Bend forward, breathing out, taking one hand to each foot/knee/shin/thigh.

7. Bring the legs back together and follow with a Seated Forward Bend (Paschimottanasana).

8. This can be repeated several times.

■ Variations

From this same legs-apart position a number of variations can be done, all of which encourage strength through the torso, good positioning of the spine and shoulders, and engagement of the pelvic floor and abdominals. These serve to improve overall strength and stability.

1. From sitting upright, gently twist, keeping the body upright and shoulders level; take the hands to the floor and bend, as if you are going to put your head on the floor to the right, and then return and go to the left.

2. Another option would be to lift the arms in an outstretched position at shoulder height, with palms together above the head, parallel in front, or holding a block. Turn the torso to the left and then to the right.

3. Place one hand on the floor beside you and reach the other up and over your head; let the spine bend to the side, going only as far as is possible. Return your arm, hand to the floor. Repeat this with the other arm.

4. Relax and ease out the knees, before moving into an easy back-bend counter-pose.

◼ Easy back-bend counter-pose

Instruction

1. From the seated position, take your arms back, hands to the floor and lean back on straight arms.

2. Inhale and arch the back, opening the chest and lifting the breastbone up. Support the neck and head by tucking the chin in slightly to engage the sternocleidomastoid. Do not let the head just loll backward.

3. Round the spine, dropping the head forward to release the neck.

4. Move from one position to the other, or, if you have more stamina and strength, hold the pose, with breathing.

Teaching focus

- Building a strong core.
- Grounding through the 'sit' bones and base of the spine.
- Muladhara and Swadhistana chakras.
- Stretching the back of the body, hamstrings and adductors.
- Pay attention to alignment for the knees and to the leg angle, and give advice as to personal adjustments, to ensure that there is no strain.

◼ Head-to-knee Forward Bend (Janu Sirsasana) (seated one-leg bend)

This is a complex posture for the average Parkinson's/MS student, but these postures offer opportunities to challenge the nerve pathways, for awareness and coordination.

To enable a correct upright seated position and without forcing the hip, use supporting blocks and/or folded blankets.

Instruction

1. With one leg in front, bend the other knee and let it rest out to the side, taking care to move the whole leg from the hip and not just forcing the knee down. Take time for the body to get used to this position and wait for the joint to ease. In older students, it is good to be kind to the joints, to give them time to release and to prepare.

2. Gently press the hand down along the thigh, and stroke down with medium pressure along the muscle, from hip to knee.

3. When the outward limit of the move is found, adjust the support. This means keeping the spine upright and placing the required number of blocks in place to support the leg near the hip joint, not directly under the knee; you can build an angle from two blocks, to suit the individual. When this is in place, the bent leg can rest against the support and release a little more. The straight leg may also need support behind the knee.

4. From this supported position you can progress to the forward-bend part of the asana, lengthening the spine and extending the arms upwards, moving up and forward over the leg, bending from the hip joint. Let the hands come down onto the leg wherever they can. Don't try to touch the toes.

Teaching focus

- Good seated posture, core engaged.
- Encourage hip releasing by using breath and visualising softness, freedom and space within the joint.
- Stretching into hamstrings and spine.
- Bring awareness into Swadhistana.

■ Revolved Side Angle Pose (Parivrtta Janu Sirsasana) (one-leg side bend)

Instruction

1. From a seated wide-leg position, bend the left knee in, supported as before. Let your right hand move down the inside of the right (straight) leg, going only as far as you can without straining.

2. When you reach your limit, turn your chest towards the left and lift the left arm up towards the ceiling. Keep the right shoulder aiming at the right knee, without turning the movement into a forward bend.

3. Hold for several breaths.

Teaching focus

- Correct and adjust the posture.
- Lateral movement of the spine, making 'space' between the vertebrae.

- Sitting into both 'sit' bones, not lifting up on one side.

- Breathing into the stretch and opening up the ribcage.

- Allowing a sense of ease to come into the posture, while holding.

■ Revolved Side Angle Pose (Parivrtta Janu Sirsasana), chair version

Instruction

1. On a chair with the knees apart, turn a little to the left and aim the right shoulder at the right knee.

2. Take the right hand to the inside of the right knee, and slide it down the inside of the leg to the ankle.

3. Lift the left arm and continue to turn the body.

4. Hold and breathe, and repeat on the other side.

■ Downward-facing Dog Pose (Ardho Muka Svanasana)

This is another good all-round posture that offers great stretch for the legs, spine and shoulders, but one that can pose a problem for those with limited mobility. I have included it here as it is classically worked from the floor, although a standing version could be offered using the wall (see page 107).

Instruction

1. Have blocks to hand and a wedge-shaped block, folded blanket and/or towel.

2. Warm up the wrists and ankles first, with 'flex and extend'. If there is pain in these joints or rigidity, offer a wedge-shaped block or folded blanket under the heels and wrists. Make sure that the toes are able to bend and support weight.

3. Begin in Cat Pose (see page 51) on hands and knees, with hands a little forward of the shoulders. Lift the knees off the ground gradually, and begin to tread the heels down alternately, to ease the hamstrings.

4. Bring the knees back to the floor for rest time, and repeat. Stay with this preliminary practice until you feel ready to explore the pose further.

5. When this has been worked, attempt to lift both knees together; lift the heels too, and then lower them gradually to the mat/support.

6. Pay attention to the shoulders, spine and hands. The hands should be actively engaged on the mat. You may like to hold a brick-shaped block rather than have the hand flat. Make sure it won't slip on the mat. Move the body towards the legs and create a hollow back as much as is possible.

7. Breathe gently but do not force the breath – breathing should be comfortable. This posture enables some 'draining' of the chest if it can be held with comfort.

8. Find when you need to stop from your own awareness.

Teaching focus

- Encourage listening to the body.

- Ground through feet and hands.

- Keep it playful and encourage the student to give up struggling.

Contraindication: This posture is really an inverted posture and is therefore not helpful for conditions such as high blood pressure, sinusitis, glaucoma and eye problems such as detached retina, nor is it suitable for acute carpel tunnel syndrome or painful arthritic feet. Shoulder problems can sometimes be a problem, but can also benefit, depending on the problem.

■ Gate Pose (Parighasana)

Gate Pose is a lateral flexion movement and provides an opportunity for stretching multiple muscle groups. This is a chair-supported version and may need additional support with rolled blankets or small soft blocks for under the feet and ankles.

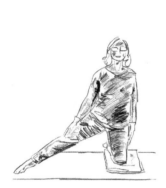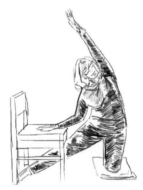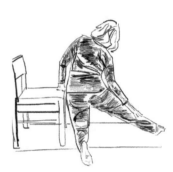

Instruction

1. Use a folded blanket placed under the knees, and place a chair in front of you, on the mat. Kneel on the mat, facing the long side.

2. Kneel on the mat, facing the long side.

3. With your knees parallel, stand up on them, so that your right hip is next to the seat of the chair. Hold the chair.

4. Stretch the left leg out to the side.

5. Keep your hips and knees in a vertical line.

6. Connect the sole of your foot into the mat. Support your foot with a rolled blanket or block, similar with the ankle of the bent leg.

7. Drop your left hand on to the left leg and slide it down towards the foot, creating a side bend for your body.

8. If you feel stable, let go of the chair and extend your right arm up towards the ceiling.

9. You can extend the stretch by reaching over and alongside your head, creating a crescent moon shape with your arms.

10. Breathe into the stretch and visualise lengthening.

11. Return by lifting the right arm up and lowering it back to the chair, bringing your spine upright.

12. Repeat on the other side.

13. Counter-pose with a forward fold such as Child Pose or a spine release such as Cat Pose (see page 51).

A variation is to hold the chair with the left hand, and to reach up and over with the right. This prevents the shoulders from twisting.

Teaching focus

- As this is a side-bending posture, check that the shoulders stay aligned on top of each other on the lateral plane, and that the spine does not twist forwards.

- Check the positioning of the neck, with the chin slightly in.

- Encourage the front of the hip joint to lengthen and open. Don't let the hips 'sit' into the ankle, even if this feels limiting.

- Work pain-free, using Ahimsa.

- Visualise the posture in your mind's eye. Hold its shape and feel it in your mind.

- Identify any tightness, breathe and visualise changes that melt tension and lengthen and soften muscles.

Parkinson's/MS note: This may take time, as it is a complex posture. In Parkinson's students, watch for the confused messaging that often occurs, and give hands-on support and encouragement, without pushing. For both groups, cramps often happen in this outstretched leg position.

Contraindication: This posture would be contraindicated for anyone with painful knees.

▣ Gate Pose from the chair

Instruction

1. Sit towards the front of the chair, with feet parallel.

2. Stretch the right leg out straight to the side.

3. Place your right hand on the leg, and begin to slide it down the leg as you exhale.

4. Inhale and lift your left arm up. Extend over to create the crescent moon shape.

5. Hold and breathe into the stretch.

6. Keep the shoulders aligned over one another, so as not to twist forwards.

7. Return, bringing your right arm down and your spine upright.

8. Repeat on the other side.

Teaching focus

- Alignment.
- Staying rooted in the 'sit' bones.
- Visualise the space between your knee, ribs and fingertips.
- Visualise the crescent shape – imagine holding a moon in your arms.
- Align the head and neck.

■ Extended Side Angle Pose (Utthita Parsvakonasana)

This posture offers the challenge of lunging, stretching, balance and strength. Use side bends, leg stretches and hip movement warm-ups.

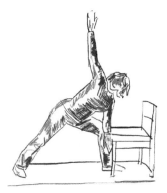 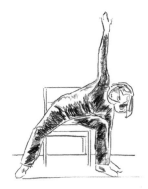

Instruction

1. Place a chair on the mat with the seat facing you.
2. Step the right foot forward to be level with the seat, so that when your knee bends, it just rests against the seat.
3. Exhale and bend the right knee at a right angle, if possible.
4. Straighten the left leg with the foot angled inwards. Connect the outside edge of the foot into the floor.
5. Lean over the right thigh and place your right forearm on the chair with the elbow just above the knee. Establish steadiness. Breathe steadily and smoothly.
6. With your left hand on your hip, align the shoulders so that they are in line and the chest turns out.
7. Raise the left arm, first up towards the ceiling, and then bring the arm over alongside the ear, to complete a full side stretch, keeping the neck long.
8. Take care to lift out in a controlled way, using the chair to push up against.

Teaching focus

- Connecting into the ground.

- Building strength in the legs.

- Muladhara – the positive aspects of this chakra are strength, courage and boldness. Bring these ideas forward.

- Take the whole posture step by step. Check that students stay within safe limits.

- Aid the alignment, guiding with words and hands.

■ Extended Side Angle Pose (Utthita Parsvakonasana), chair version

Instruction

1. Sit to the front of the chair and perch the 'sit' bones firmly near the edge.

2. Turn the right knee out as far as possible, with the foot firmly on the floor.

3. Open your hips and stretch the left leg straight. Place the sole of the foot on the floor.

4. Place your right elbow on the right knee.

5. Turn the trunk to the front.

6. Inhale and extend the left arm up and then over alongside your ear. Point the fingers away.

7. For a deeper experience, place a block or two by your right foot, and lean over the right thigh, connecting your body to your thigh.

8. Reach your right hand down to the block, knee tucked under your armpit.

9. Complete the left arm stretch.

10. Push against the floor to lift out of the posture, or walk your hands up your leg.

Teaching focus

- Adjust the practice according to the mobility and fitness of your students.

■ Reclining Hand-to-Big-Toe Pose (Supta Padangusthasana)

This is great for tight hamstrings, and useful practice before some of the forward bends.

You will need a strap, a block for under the head and a rolled blanket to be placed under the straight knee.

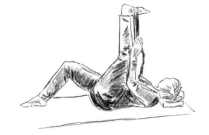

Instruction

1. Lie on the mat in a straight line.

2. Bend the right leg and place a strap around the foot. Keep the left leg straight (with the rolled blanket behind the knee).

3. Hold the strap with both hands and straighten the leg as far as possible.

4. Hold the position, firm and steady. Breathe smoothly.

5. Draw the leg a little closer to increase the stretch – explore what is possible, but do not strain.

6. Further the asana by resting the left hand on the hip to stop the pelvis from rolling, at the same time opening the right leg out to the right sideways. Keep both legs stretched.

7. Work still further by holding the strap with the left hand, right hand on hip, and taking the right leg across the body.

Teaching focus

- Activating the core muscles will enable this posture to be held steadily without rolling to facilitate better lengthening in the legs.

- Observe the students to assist with steadiness.

Reclining Hand-to-Big-Toe Pose (Supta Padangusthasana), chair version

Instruction

A chair can be used in various ways:

1. Stand with your right foot on the chair seat, with your leg straight. Loop the strap around your foot. Explore holding the strap in both hands and bend towards the straight leg.

2. Hold the strap in your right hand and turn your body away from the stretched leg, opening out the left hand as you do so.

3. Hold the strap in your left hand and turn to the right.

4. Sit on the chair, fold the right knee in, loop the strap round the right foot, holding the strap in both hands, like reins. Stretch out the leg and use the strap to lift it higher.

5. Hold the strap in the right hand and turn the body to the left.

6. Hold the strap in the left hand and turn the body to the right.

7. Follow this stretch by bending the knees in, one at a time.

Parkinson's/MS note: Almost all of the students I have ever had in class love stretching with the strap as it eases spasms, cramps and rigidity.

Restorative practices

Restorative yoga is a passive supported form of yoga allowing the student to rest deeply while the body yields into the posture. For most people, restorative postures help to balance and restore energy flow (Lasater 2011). However, for the two groups of students that we are considering here, the experience will be different. While helpful in counteracting postural problems and easing out stiff joints, there are some aspects of these held postures that prove difficult, for those with Parkinson's especially.

These postures will need to be offered as one-to-one Yoga Therapy sessions, as you will need to observe your student closely. Their posture, spine shape, joint positioning and level of comfort will all be factors to consider in adjustments. Choose the simpler practices, and note the props needed. These postures may not be possible if people are severely immobile. Getting down into the positions and moving on the floor may be a challenge, and holding for any length of time often increases discomfort, spasm and cramping, thereby undoing any of the positive effects.

I would not recommend:

- Supported bound angle: This is too restricting for most people with Parkinson's, and causes spasm and cramps after time, even when well supported. Students who have tried this found they were not able to remain comfortable and began to feel pain.

- Supported forward bend: Practising this on the floor with a bolster in front proves nigh on impossible for most people with Parkinson's. It works much better using a chair or ball to support. Tight adductors and stiff spines prevent a comfortably held pose that can encourage release.

The following work well – students enjoyed them, and found that they could practise at home.

■ Fish Pose (Matsyasana) (supported back bend)

Plan to allow one minute in the pose and gradually increase the time.

Instruction

1. You will need a block, rolled blanket or bolster. The head and neck will need support, so have an extra block or rolled blanket ready.

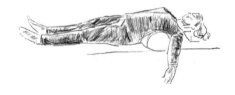

2. Start in semi-supine, and begin very simply, with just one block under the shoulder blades to let the spine ease over the support.

3. Keep the neck free from pressure and allow it to lengthen away. Use more support if needed. The shoulders should be on or near the floor (check that the back arch position is not over-contracted and adjust the support if necessary).

4. The teacher will help you to come out of the posture by helping you to roll over sideways; then sit up slowly.

5. Depending on your flexibility and spinal shape and length, a bolster can be used instead of a block, to increase the arch. The bolster or a firm rolled blanket can be placed so that it supports the thoracic spine.

The posture should not be painful – it should be more of a restful stretch. It is a very useful restorative practice for helping Parkinson's and MS students who suffer from spinal rigidity and postural problems, and is useful for counteracting rolled-in 'round' shoulders and a slumped posture, tight pectoral muscles and shoulder joints.

Contraindication: Be especially mindful of lordosis and severe kyphosis. This posture would be contraindicated for spondylitis or degenerative disc disease. Care may be needed with shoulder joint problems, but it can help to unwind tightness in a recovering frozen shoulder.

Energy and emotional awareness: This posture is a heart-opening posture, and it puts the practitioner in an open and vulnerable position. This may open up possibilities to explore how it feels to:

- be exposed
- face a fear
- open the heart – Anahata chakra
- surrender.

■ Supported twist

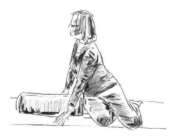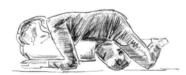

Allow two minutes on each side for this pose.

Instruction

1. You will need a bolster and a folded blanket, and possibly an extra blanket. Sit with the right hip close to the end of the bolster, with knees bent and feet to the left.

2. Turn towards the bolster and lift and lengthen your spine before leaning over onto the bolster, with hands placed either side, lengthening the torso on lowering down. Turn the head to one side into a comfortable resting position.

3. Make sure that your hands and head are comfortable, and use breath to ease further into the posture – go carefully and work without strain. (The teacher will cover you if you get cold.)

4. To come out of the posture, the teacher will help you to press your hands into the floor to come up.

This posture is useful for those with postural problems such as one hip higher than the other, or where there is imbalance in the quadratus and psoas muscles, and for the spine, although caution is needed with severe back problems. The height of the support may need to be adjusted if there is a chronic limitation. The head and neck may need careful support until a comfortable position is found. This can be a difficult area for Parkinson's. This posture is safe for most people, but always check with your student how they are experiencing the posture.

Energy and emotional awareness:

- Be aware of the energy flow along the spine, and which areas are most rotated.

- Focus on bringing space and openness into the lumbar and mid thoracic areas.

- Explore feeling safe and resting deeply.

■ Supported Child's Pose (Balasana)

Allow three minutes for time in the pose.

Instruction

1. You will need a bolster, a folded blanket, two rolled towels and a sandbag (this is optional).

2. With a folded blanket on the mat and the bolster longways, kneel, with your knees hip-width apart, with the bolster in front.

3. The feet should be pointed back and a rolled towel placed under the ankles for support.

4. Another towel can be placed behind the knees if you find it uncomfortable to hold the deep bend.

5. Move the bolster between the thighs.

6. Lengthen your body along the bolster (the sandbag can be placed on the lower back to enhance relaxation of the muscles).

7. Breathing should be unrestricted; move the bolster to give more space if needed.

8. The tailbone should drop towards the floor.

9. Take time positioning the head to one side and support it to give comfort; this can be moved after a little time.

10. The arms go back towards the feet or rest in front. Rest in the posture.

11. To come out of the pose, press your hands to the floor to push up, and then come out of the kneeling position. (The teacher will give help if you need it. They may need to bring your feet to one side and then around so you are back in a comfortable sitting position.) Do some straight leg stretches before transferring to a chair.

This posture gently stretches the lower back, relieves shoulder tension and quietens the mind.

Teaching focus

- With permission, there could be hands-on help to the lower back or tight shoulders. This would provide warmth and comfort, encouraging awareness in these often-tight areas, and encouraging release. Do not massage (unless you are qualified and insured to do so).

Contraindication: If there are varicose veins, compression in the legs is contraindicated. This can be accommodated by using more support to lift the hips by sitting on a block, for example, to relieve the pressure. If the breathing feels inhibited – for instance, if the person carries weight on the breasts or stomach – create more lift for the chest and space for the stomach. Offer a chair version.

■ Supported Child's Pose (Balasana), chair-supported version

Instruction

1. Sit on a chair, feet apart, with another chair in front.

2. A bolster should be placed on the chair in front, longways.

3. Lean forwards over the bolster, letting your arms hang loosely or letting them rest on the chair.

4. Place your head to one side, with support from a cushion or small block.

Energy and emotional awareness: Direct the breath into the back of the body, opening the back of the heart chakra, feeling into the stretch along the spine. This posture is comforting, and promotes feelings of safety and security. Work with affirmations such as 'I am safe and secure'. This may be helpful for students for whom this is an issue. It may bring forward insights into their underlying feelings.

■ Elevated legs up the wall

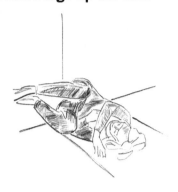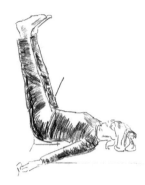

Allow 15 minutes for time in the posture.

Instruction

1. You will need a bolster, a folded blanket and a block. On the mat, with the blanket folded on top, sit close to the wall with your legs bent. The teacher may help you to roll onto your back. Take your legs up the wall.

2. If you are able, with bent knees and feet on the wall, press into the wall and lift your hips enough for the teacher to slide a bolster underneath.

3. Move the bolster away from the wall if the backs of the legs are too tight.

4. Place a folded and rolled towel under the base of the neck to preserve its natural curve.

5. The arms can then rest by the sides or above the head.

6. The teacher will help you out of the pose, by helping you to bend your knees and press your feet into the wall, and pulling the bolster away. Roll on to your side and pause, before pushing up into a sitting position.

This posture is truly restorative in that it brings blood flow to the neck and head, and rests the legs, aiding lymph flow. It is good for varicose veins, both in the legs and rectum, and will take pressure from any prolapsed conditions in the abdomen.

Caution and contraindication: This pose is not recommended for anyone who should avoid inversions – if there is hiatus hernia, eye pressure problems or detached retina or other retinal problems, heart problems, neck problems or menstruation (optional, if periods are very light). Be aware of any discomfort in the lower back. It should not be used for those with high blood pressure, but may be used if the condition is medicated. Avoid it if there is a sinus infection or head cold, or an inflamed ear condition. Where there is a kyphotic spine, this may prove too uncomfortable to be restful, unless you can provide support with more folded blankets.

Energy and emotional awareness:

- Vishuddhi, Ajna, Sahasrara chakras.

- Helpful for calming the mind.

- For balancing Udana vayu and promoting Prana vayu (upward flowing energy).

- Imagine the mind emptying and 'busyness' being absorbed into the earth.

These restorative practices will vary greatly with each individual. Some may need a lot of support and 'handling' to help them in and out of positions. Always explain what you are going to do and demonstrate how to move and be in the posture, how you will adapt and support, and ask for permission to aid them. It is helpful if they have a helper with them who is used to helping them to move and get up and down.

■ Relaxation postures

Supporting the body for relaxation is both helpful and comforting.

Instruction

1. You will need two or three blankets, a bolster and a block. The blanket should be folded and placed on the mat, either under the whole of the spine or under the hips. This is especially good for students who have little flesh covering – a blanket will cushion the boney places.

2. Place a block under the head to keep the back of the neck long and free.

3. Place a bolster or thick rolled blanket under the knees.

4. Other helpful additions could be an eye pillow, which gives a soothing weight to the eyelids.

5. Cover the feet for warmth if required, and add a blanket to cover the whole body.

6. Elevating the legs for relaxation is also an excellent way of relieving tiredness and aiding lymph drainage: a chair should be placed on the mat, with a folded blanket over the seat of the chair to provide cushioning. Lift your legs onto the chair seat, adjusting for height.

7. In this position students can be guided into relaxation with a focus on soothing breath and appropriate visualisation, or yoga nidra to induce deep rest.

THERAPEUTIC MUDRA

According to Swami Satyananda Saraswati:

> Mudra practices establish a direct link between Annamaya Kosha, Manomaya Kosha and Pranamaya Kosha. Mudras manipulate prana in much the same way that energy in the form of light or sound waves is diverted by a mirror or a cliff face. The nadis and chakras constantly radiate prana which normally escapes from the body and dissipates into the external world. By creating barriers within the body through the practice of Mudra, the energy is redirected within.

A small study in 2008 by Heather Blashki of the Australian Institute of Yoga Therapy showed some effectiveness in using hasta mudras (yoga hand gestures) for some common ailments. The main research question for this study was: 'Will regular practice of hasta mudras reduce symptoms or relieve pain in specific health conditions?' The results found that there was a 20.6 per cent reduction in pain or symptom levels in the test group compared with an 8.9 per cent reduction in the control group. Anxiety was reduced by 20.5 per cent in the test group and by 12.2 per cent in the control group, stress (reduced) by 17.2 per cent in the test group and 8.8 per cent in the control group. There was a statistically significant change in the mood level of the test groups, with an improvement (increased calmness) of 28.6 per cent compared with a deterioration (increased irritation) of 1.6 per cent for the control group. Sleep was also (statistically) significantly improved in the test group (19 per cent) compared with a control group sleep deterioration of 6.8 per cent.

I taught these mudras to my Parkinson's students and suggested that they might experiment with them. The mudras suggested for back pain, joint pain and exhaustion proved to be useful and had a positive, albeit temporary, effect.

I have included these as supportive and restorative practices. They can be practised at any time, even when watching TV, and do not need particular focus. However, some people may find them impossible if they have spasm, spasticity or arthritis in the fingers.

■ Joint pain mudra

To relieve joint pain and inflammation.

Instruction

1. Right hand: bring the tips of the thumb and third finger together.

2. Left hand: bring together the tip of the thumb and the second finger.

■ Back pain mudra

Instruction

1. Right hand: Let the tip of the forefinger touch the crease of the joint of the thumb.

2. Left hand: Join the tip of the thumb, the second finger and little finger.

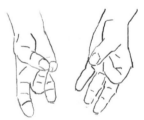

■ Pran mudra

Instruction

For tiredness and exhaustion:

1. Both hands: Bring the tip of the thumb, ring finger and little finger together.

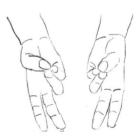

Digestion

It is important to follow the specific guidelines for diet that work with the drug regime for optimal absorption of any medicines prescribed. A balanced diet that keeps the body at a healthy weight is dependent on the intestinal tract working efficiently. Unfortunately, in both Parkinson's and MS, the disease process affects the muscular movement of the digestive tract, which can lead to chronic constipation. There may also be increased anxiety around eating as slowness of movement prolongs mealtimes, and food becomes unappetisingly cold. Tremor impairs manual dexterity and adds to the difficulties. Some people with Parkinson's find they are not eating enough. These factors mean that the process of digestion is slow and there is a sluggish uptake of nutrients. Stimulating the action of peristalsis and assisting the movement of food through the gut is therefore of great benefit.

If there are concerns regarding overall nutrition, however, refer the patient to a suitably qualified nutrition expert.

The five movements commonly worked in Laghoo Shankaprakshalana (intestinal cleansing) really help to stretch and move the intestinal tract. These can be offered as a sequence of standing postures and can be adapted for a chair, bearing in mind that this will limit the full action. Full Laghoo Shankaprakshalana (intestinal cleansing) is not suitable for Parkinson's or MS, unless there is medical supervision, as the action and effect with medication is not known.

◼ The five stretches

Instruction

1. Stretch 1: Vertical stretching. Stand with the feet parallel and stretch the arms upwards as you inhale and lower them on exhaling. Repeat this five times. This can be done smoothly and quickly or a little slower as preferred. Feel this stretch along the front of the body.

2. Stretch 2: Side stretching. Clasp your hands and raise your arms; sway from side to side. Be aware of the stretch through the sides of the body. Repeat five times (ten moves).

These first two stretches begin to move the upper section of the digestive tract.

3. Stretch 3: Twisting. Twisting postures have a powerful action and really get the system moving. This is a rhythmic and loose twist. Turn the whole body from the shoulders and let the arms twist naturally around the body, left hand to rest near the right hip and right to left. Repeat five times (ten moves).

All of these can be done from a chair, making sure that there is lengthening through the torso.

4. Stretch 4: Lying face down with hands under the shoulders. Using a rolling movement, press down with the left hand and look over the right shoulder. Return, and press down with the right hand and look over the left shoulder. This

creates a rolling action on the abdomen, making a massage action for the lower part of the digestive tract.

There are ways to recreate this movement from other positions according to the needs of the student and what support is available. For example, if it is impossible to lie on the floor, try this sitting option. Sit up on the 'sit' bones and bend forward to rest your body along your legs; hold the chair with the hands next to the knees. Slide the right hand onto the hip and turn the body to the right, lifting the top shoulder up. This creates a similar rolling action on the abdomen. Move back to the legs and roll the other way, sliding the left hand onto the hip.

It may be also be possible to create this abdominal massage by kneeling and resting over a chair. Kneel and bend forward over a chair, bring your arms behind your back and lift the right shoulder turning the body, as if you are going to look over your shoulder, and then repeat on the other side.

Or, if kneeling is impossible, a similar action can be created by standing with your body pressed against a wall. Place your hands on the wall under the shoulders and create the lift and turn. The abdomen in contact with the wall provides a massage action. This is not as powerful as the kneeling or lying version, though, as it does not have the same pressure.

5. Stretch 5: Crow. This final move is a challenge even for the practised, able-bodied person, and would be too much for most people with Parkinson's and MS. But the action is one of twisting and creating pressure in the ascending and descending colons. The easiest way to apply this for those unable to get into a deep squat is on a chair. Bend one knee up and hug it close in until you can get your heel on the chair seat, or just as far as is possible. Keep it pulled in close and turn in towards the knee, creating a deep compression in the abdomen. Release and place the feet back on the floor, and then draw up the other knee and repeat on the other side. Do this five times on each side.

Twisting postures always have a good deep massaging action on the digestive system. These postures also have many other beneficial applications. There are a number of ways in which they can be offered, according to the fitness and ability of the students, and a number of modifications can be offered.

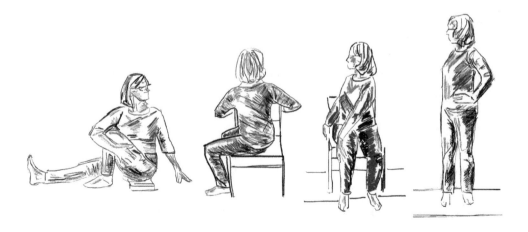

◼ Modified Sage Pose (Marichyasana) (seated twist)

A seated twist will have gravity working alongside the pressure and massage action of the posture to aid peristalsis, enabling more efficient movement of food through the system (in yoga terms, improved Apana flow and therefore elimination). Manipura chakra is stimulated and energised. This asana may be contraindicated for some types of hip replacement (the full joint type).

Instruction

1. From the supported sitting position on the floor, using blocks under the 'sit' bones, draw up the right knee and place the right foot next to the left knee; hold on to the knee with both hands, draw the spine up and sit up.

2. Hold on to the knee with the left hand, and extend the right hand forward at shoulder height.

3. Turn towards the knee, drawing it as close to the body as possible, as you sweep the right arm around to the back, placing that hand on the ground or on a block or perched on fingertips.

4. Continue the spinal twist by letting the head and neck join in the movement to look back over the shoulder. Use the eye muscles as well. Hold, and breathe in, encouraging a little more turn on the out-breath.

5. Return and repeat with the left knee bent and right leg straight.

To further the twist:

6. Bring the right knee closer to the body, cross the right foot over the left knee and repeat the twist with the same instruction, focus and guidance.

7. The object of the practice is not achievement of the full posture, but enough to bring health benefits with the knee as close to the body as possible to create pressure in the colon.

8. Hold and breathe and repeat on the other side.

◼ Modified Sage Pose (Marichyasana), wall version

There two ways to use the wall for support, sitting and standing.

Instruction

Sitting instructions:

1. Place the mat alongside the wall, with a block to sit on.

2. Sit up tall in Staff Pose (Dandasana) (see page 60), with the right side against the wall, and bend the right leg up as near to the body as possible and inhale.

3. Hold the knee and lengthen the trunk upwards.

4. Exhale and turn towards the wall, using your hands against the wall to aid the turn. You can also press the left elbow against the right knee.

5. Repeat facing the other way to work the other side.

Standing instructions:

1. Place a chair against the wall, sideways on.

2. Put your right foot onto the chair seat.

3. Lengthen your spine upwards and inhale.

4. Exhale and turn towards the wall.

5. Use your hands against the wall to steady the position.

Teaching focus

*   The spine should remain upright, and not slump back, even if this means a less strong turn.

*   Encourage releasing and turning on the out-breath.

*   Encourage the placement of the abdomen against the leg, feeling the breath in the belly creating a massage action.

*   Energising Manipura chakra.

*   Gentle hands-on assistance by guiding the spine upwards and enhancing the turn.

Lying twist

The twisting action of this posture will provide a massage action on the gut to encourage movement. This posture will support Samana vayu and activate the energies of Manipura chakra at the level of Annamaya kosha. If we are trying to stimulate the digestive tract, we can use a more moving version of the posture and encourage slow repeats, while maintaining the stretch.

There are stages in applying this asana. We begin with the easiest.

■ Semi-supine twist

Instruction

1. Lying with the knees bent and head supported, so that the neck is aligned, and depending on space, stretch the arms out along the floor at shoulder level. If there is not room to do this, have the elbows bent, with the arms cupping the back of the head.

2. Take the knees part of the way to the left, on an exhale breath. Moving to the left first exerts a little pressure on the rising colon and works the body in a way that optimises the passage of food through the digestive tract.

3. Bring the legs back to the centre on an inhale breath, and take them over to the right, exhaling.

4. This can be repeated two or three times, gradually increasing the twisting action until the legs are going as far over as is possible within a pain-free range. The shoulders should stay on the floor so that the upper body is stable. Head turning can be added to complete the twist action, but only if you are comfortable with this.

5. Once the posture becomes familiar, you can hold for longer, with gentle normal breathing, allowing time for release in the joints and muscles. During the time the posture is held, visualise the muscle lengthening and softness spreading through tight areas, visualising Samana vayu as warmth spreading around the stomach area.

6. Come out of the posture when you are ready (this encourages awareness).

Teaching focus

- Alignment of the spine, head and neck; the shoulders stay on the floor.

- Massage action on the digestive tract.

- Focus on Manipura.

- Explain the action of Samana vayu and warmth moving in a circular action around the navel.

- Offer gentle hands-on assistance in keeping steady and improving the turn.

Parkinson's note: It may be difficult for some to move very far because of rigidity in the spine. Support may be needed with a folded blanket under the back.

The following variations may offer slightly different actions:

1. Offer a block to be held between the knees, and encourage squeezing it on the turn, focusing on the adductors, and encourage engagement of the pelvic floor.

2. A harder option is to slide the left leg straight and take the right leg over and across the body. This may require a pile of blocks to support the knee and to take the strain. This also offers an opportunity for hands-on easing, if the student is comfortable with that. Place one hand on the shoulder, but do not force; just aid the student in keeping it in place. The other hand can help the hip, giving a diagonal stretch. Do this incrementally, with the student's permission.

■ One-Leg Forward Bend (Janu Sirsasana)

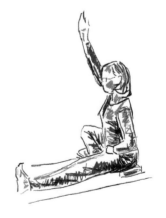

This version is designed to deeply massage the colon. To enable a correct upright seated position and without forcing the hip, use supporting blocks and/or folded blankets. The right side must be worked first to exert a massage action in the ascending colon and ileocecal valve.

Instruction

1. With the right leg straight, bend the left knee and rock it out to the side, taking care to move the whole leg from the hip and not just force the knee down. Take time for the body to get used to this position and wait for the joint to ease. In older students, it is good to be kind to the joints, to give them time to release and prepare.

2. Gently press the hand down along the thigh, and stroke down with medium pressure along the muscle from the hip to the knee.

3. When the outward limit of the move is found, adjust the support. This means keeping the spine upright and placing the required number of blocks in place to support the leg near the hip joint, not directly under the knee; you can build an angle from two blocks, to suit the individual. When this is in place, the bent leg can rest against the support and you may be able to release a little more. The straight leg may also need supporting behind the knee.

4. From this supported position you can progress to the forward-bend part of the asana. Place your right fist in the right groin, or a rolled blanket or towel to create a gentle pressure.

5. Lengthen the spine upwards and extend the left arm to move up and forward over the leg, bending from the hip joint.

6. Let the hand come down onto the leg wherever it can, but do not try to touch the toes. If the body is able to move this far, you will be pressing on to the fist.

7. Hold for a slow count of ten. Release the bend and the pressure, and come up.

8. Do this on the other side with the left leg straight and the left hand in a fist in the left groin, to exert pressure on the descending colon.

Teaching focus

- Creating a deep massage action to aid the movement of waste products through the colon.

- This action stimulates Apana.

- Bring awareness into Muladhara chakra.

- Counter-pose with a gentle seated back bend.

Contraindication: Stop if there is pain. Do not do this if there is any inflamed condition, irritable bowel or grumbling appendix.

■ Upward Abdominal Lift (Uddiyana Bhanda)

This is a dynamic practice that can be useful because of its strong action around the diaphragm. It will stimulate Samana and ignite the digestive 'fire'. Use cautiously: check for any hernia, other inflammatory abdominal condition or heart problems.

Instruction

1. Stand in a semi-stooped position and rest your hands on the insides of your knees. Let the back be rounded.

2. Inhale deeply and exhale.

3. Hold empty. Draw the abdomen in and out sharply five times.

4. Breathe in.

5. Repeat, and gradually build up the number of abdominal contractions.

Teaching focus

- This must be practised cautiously – it is likely to be more useful to MS students and those who are able, fit and well.

■ Apanasana

This is a good resting posture in between some of the more strenuous work, but also provides compression and release in the abdomen, creating a massage action. Work the preliminary one-leg folds first, and go with the flow of food in the system by pulling the right leg in first. Hold with both legs folded to focus on the breath and massage action. This is a relaxing action that will also help to facilitate good digestion.

Instruction

1. Lie flat on the floor in semi-supine. Support the head with a block to keep a length in the neck.

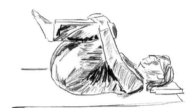

2. Bend the right knee, reach and clasp it in your hands and fold it towards your body, as you exhale.

3. Hug the knee in towards your chest and inhale.

4. Exhale and lift your head up towards your knee.

5. Inhale and put your head back on the block, exhale and lift it towards the knee. Repeat this action five times.

6. Slide the leg away, and draw the left leg in.

7. Repeat the movements and breathing.

8. Draw both knees up together and hug them in. Breathe in and out, and allow the action of the breath in the diaphragm to move the legs away. This should not be forced in any way.

Teaching focus

- Check for the head/neck position and support where needed.

- Imagine breathing into the abdomen and lower back.

- Stimulating Apana.

Chair work

In this section we will explore the possibilities of modifying asana for those who are unable to stand without support. It includes sitting postures and some chair-supported versions of classical asana.

■ Sitting Mountain Pose

If your students are unable to stand, use the same focus to direct chair Mountain Pose (Tadasana) (see page 78). Encourage good posture, sitting 'up' on the 'sit' bones, maintaining the lower curve of the back, feet and knees hip-width apart. The feet can be placed on a block. Keep alignment awareness active. This means:

- Keep in parallel alignment.
- Keep grounding through the feet and tailbone.
- Pay attention to the position of the shoulders.
- Pay attention to the position of head and neck.
- The chest should be open.
- Activate the core muscles.
- Maintain length through the whole of the spine.
- Breathe along the spine, up from the feet. Spread the breath into and around the ribcage.
- Sitting Mountain Pose is a good starting point for many postures.

Teaching focus

- Check that the students are not slumping in the chair.
- Use light 'hands-on' guidance to encourage lift through the spine and chest and to move the shoulders down.
- It may be useful to use a cushion or pillow to support a more upright posture in the chair.

SITTING WARM-UPS

All of the 'joint freeing' for the neck, arms and hands and feet detailed in the preliminaries can be worked as warm-ups for all of the chair yoga (see pages 41–49).

■ Undulating to warm up the spine

Instruction

1. Sit upright on the 'sit' bones.

2. Begin exhaling with a hollowing of the abdomen, rounding the back and drawing the abdominal muscles in.

3. Arch the back, opening the chest, and breathe in. Let the movement flow from one action to the opposite.

4. Feel into the movement and notice any areas that are not moving or that feel stuck.

5. Focus on letting the movement begin from the stuck place, and keep the spine moving into a 'C' shape, back and forth.

6. Further movement awareness can be encouraged by moving from the 'C' shape into an 'S' shape.

Teaching focus

• Allow the group to play with this free-form flowing movement.

• Explore the restrictions and keep the movements flowing.

• The whole spine is energised during this process – the joints, muscles and fascia get a workout.

• As everyone is working within their own parameters, there are few contraindications to this flowing warm-up.

■ Seated side bend

Many yoga teachers are familiar with this stretch that lengthens through the latissimus dorsi and opens up the intercostal muscles. In this position we can encourage breathing coordination.

In a chair it is important to assess whether the students can maintain balance while doing side movements. Side bends are done more safely by holding the chair with one or both arms, while exploring the movement of the spine.

Instruction

1. Have the knees apart, feet firmly down. Use blocks under the feet if this helps to ground.

2. Engage the core muscles to provide a strong base.

3. Hold the chair with your left hand and on the inhale breath stretch the right arm up.

4. Exhale, bending to the left, and extend the lifted arm alongside the head. Lengthen away to the fingertips.

5. Keep the feet and legs steady without losing grounding.

6. Hold and breathe. You can progress the posture and encourage stamina by adding more breath repetitions on the hold.

7. Come back to upright and lower the arm, exhaling and relaxing.

8. Repeat on the other side.

Teaching focus

- Check for any limitation in shoulder extension, and keep the focus on the movement of the spine rather than the lift of the arms.

- If there is shoulder injury, frozen shoulder or severe kyphosis, the movement will be limited. Check that there is no forcing through any joint that is limited in this way.

- If there is pain in any movement, encourage working within the pain-free range.

- It is important to engage the core muscles, to promote inner strength and good posture.

- Make sure the spine is not twisting forward or back.

- 'Earthing' through the base chakra.

- Stimulates Apana through grounding and Vyana through the arm action.

- Bring awareness into the opening of the ribcage and breathe into the open ribs.

- This posture gives the teacher an opportunity to guide gently with a hand on the shoulder using words to encourage, rather than pulling or pushing. Light touch and gentle instruction are enough to bring attention to the posture and encourage stretching and opening.

- We can remind the body how it needs to adjust even if we repeat the same instructions week by week.

- Extra attention can be given where there is rigidity, muscle spasm and immobility.

Bear in mind that in an older population the spine may already be changing its shape and its curves, and make allowances for this. If the student has sufficient strength and stability, they can try the Swaying Palm version (see page 78), by lifting both arms in parallel. Ensure they stay anchored through the 'sit' bones.

■ Chair adaptations for sitting forward bends

If the students are not able to easily transfer up and down from the floor, there are some options for bending from the chair. Blocks can be placed under the feet for those who find it difficult to connect fully with the feet on the floor.

Seated Forward Bend (Paschimottanasana) from the chair is the same as chair Standing Forward Bend (Uttanasana). Although this does not give the same leg stretch, it will assist in keeping the spine flexible and help with muscle rigidity and strength.

Instruction

1. With the feet parallel and placed on blocks if that helps the feet to feel grounded, lift the arms in parallel, and lengthen the torso and the spine.

2. Forward bend from the hips on the exhale breath. Move into the bend slowly, going all the way down, hands to feet, or as far as they will go.

3. To progress, work this posture more slowly, stopping halfway with the spine and arms horizontal with the floor. Inhale and exhale on bending further.

4. To come out of the posture, lift and extend the arms up and forwards first, creating a horizontal line with the arms and the spine.

5. Lift all the way up and then relax.

6. If this is too strenuous, the spine can be lifted with the arms in a soft relaxed position.

A chair version of Seated Forward Bend (Paschimottanasana) can be offered with two chairs, as long as balance can be maintained. This is suitable for those who find transferring too hard, but is best with individual guidance and attention. With both legs up on the chair in front, the student can be guided into the forward fold as directed for the floor (see page 160).

■ Wide-leg variation

Instruction

1. Sit with the legs wide, knees in line with the feet. Avoid turning the knees inwards.

2. Turn the trunk towards the right knee, and lean back a little way with the core muscles engaged. Breathe in, stretch up, lift and lengthen the spine and bend from the hip over the right thigh.

3. There are then a couple of options depending on the strength of the students: Keep the stretched-out long spine position, and hold for a couple of breaths, or immediately release over the legs hands down onto the floor, before lifting out and coming back up.

4. Repeat over the other leg.

■ Revolved Head-to-Knee Pose (Parivrtta Janu Sirsasana) (wide-leg side bend)

Instruction

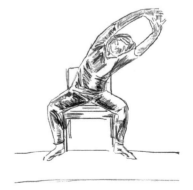

1. From the wide-leg seated position, knees aligned with the feet, turn the trunk to the left, to point the right shoulder at the right knee.

2. Lift both arms, palms facing each other, or the right hand holding the left wrist.

3. Extend over the right thigh.

4. Keep both 'sit' bones on the chair and ease as far into the side stretch as possible.

5. Return in a controlled way, lifting away and up.

6. Repeat on the other side.

Teaching focus

- Feel into the long space between the hip and the ribs, and breathe into this space.

- Visualise stretching like elastic.

- Use core strength to stabilise the posture, and stay rooted through the 'sit' bones and the feet.

■ Wide-leg, rotation and forward bend sequence, in stages

This is a sequence of movements that will work the spine, shoulders and the hips, and is a useful warm-up for further twisting and bending postures. It builds on the previous postures.

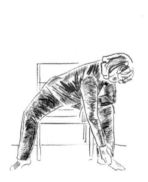 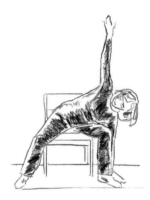

Instruction

1. To warm up, sit on the chair with the knees and feet wide, sitting up on the 'sit' bones. Place the right elbow on the right knee and drop the left hand to the right ankle.

2. Sweep the left hand out and up, turning the body and shoulders on an in-breath.

3. Breathe out and return to the start. Repeat five times on each side.

■ Stretch further

Instruction

1. Turn the body and lean over to bring the left elbow on to the right knee.

2. Place the right hand beside the right foot, or modify for stiff immobile shoulders by placing the right hand on the right hip.

3. Inhale and begin to turn from the centre of the breastbone as you lift your right arm out to shoulder height. Turn your body as far as you can comfortably go, without straining.

4. Return to the start position.

■ Extend the rotation

Instruction

1. In the wide-leg seated position, turn your body towards your right knee.

2. Lean over until your body is lying down along your thigh.

3. Let both arms come down so that your hands are on your ankle.

4. Breathe out and on the inhale lift your left arm out to shoulder height.

5. Pause and exhale.

6. Inhale and turn from the centre of the breastbone and see how far you can go without over-extending the shoulder.

7. Return, hand to foot on the exhale breath.

8. Repeat four times.

9. Repeat the same process, lifting the right hand. Internal rotation is usually easier than external rotation.

10. Repeat over the left leg.

Teaching focus

- Turn the spine rather than moving the arms so that the turn originates from the thoracic spine rather than the waist and hips.

- Modify the arm position for frozen shoulders. A hand on the hip with elbow bent will help to ensure that the spinal turn is emphasised.

- Work within personal limitations.

- Breath coordination.

- Manipura and Muladhara chakras.

- Good stable foot position, grounding and Apana.

- Breathe along the spine, following the gentle twist – imagine energy radiating outwards.

■ Intense Side Stretch Pose (Parsvottanasana) (seated One-Leg Forward Bend)

A strap and a block can be used to support this posture.

Instruction

1. Sit towards the front of the chair, and make sure you are sitting up on the 'sit' bones.

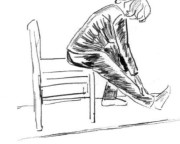

2. Stretch one leg out in front. This can be supported by putting your foot on a block (two blocks will make it harder).

3. Place your hands first on the hip joint, to become aware that this is where the movement will start. If using a strap, loop it around you foot, draping the ends over your leg.

4. Inhale and lift and lengthen upwards, and begin to lean forward from the hip joint.

5. Take both hands onto the thigh of the straight leg, and, keeping the spine long and straight, slide your hands down towards the knee and further if possible. Catch hold of the strap.

6. Let the spine stay long and keep the stretch in the hamstrings. Let the knee bend if that is more comfortable.

7. Go as far as possible and hold at the end of the stretch with steady breathing.

8. Return to upright and repeat on the other leg.

Teaching focus

- Work within personal limits. It is important not to strain. Ahimsa.

- Grounding and balance.

- Breathe into the stretch and visualise the muscles lengthening.

Two chairs can also be used as an adaptation for the one-leg stretch, by simply putting one leg up on the chair in front to stretch over.

For a counter-pose, offer a mild back bend with arms on the back of the chair seat, chest lifted, neck supported by gently tucking the chin in, arching the spine.

■ Head-to-Knee Forward Bend (Janu Sirsasana), with chair

Instruction

1. Sit well back in the chair.

2. Bend and lift the left knee, let it open out to the side and place the left foot on the right knee. Alternatively, keeping the foot on the floor, let the bent leg turn out from the hip, so that the outside edge of the foot rests on the floor (or block).

3. Lift your arms up and lengthen your spine, lean forwards, keeping the line of your arms and spine.

4. Return upright and release the left foot to the floor.

5. Repeat on the other leg.

6. It may be possible to experiment with straightening the right leg, depending on your ability.

Teaching focus

- The first version described will be a challenge for those with stiff hips, and may need caution in knee care.

- Adjustments in expectations will be essential for positive practice.

- Focus on hip releasing no matter what the level of mobility.

■ Chair back bend

Instruction

1. Sit tall towards the front of the chair, feet and knees parallel. Hold the back of the chair seat and anchor your tailbone down, as if you are growing it towards the floor.

2. Begin your back bend from the very base of the spine. Lift the spine up and the breastbone forward.

3. Support the head and neck, by tucking the chin in a little and lengthening the back of the neck. Keep the chest open and hold for four breaths.

4. Come up and release the head and neck forward.

Teaching focus

- Keep the breastbone lifted.

- Make allowances for kyphosis.

- Encourage the bend through the whole of the spine.

- Enjoy the release following the posture.

- Anahata – heart-centred energy focus.

■ Seated Warrior Pose 1

Instruction

1. Steadying yourself with your arms, sit to the front of the chair and turn to the left side so that the right 'sit' bone is off the chair.

2. Drop the right knee down towards the floor, toes tucked under.

3. Turn your torso further, so that your hips are square to the left.

4. Slide the right leg back as far as it will go, and anchor your foot to the floor, connecting through the outside edge.

5. Check for steadiness.

6. Engage the core.

7. Both arms can be lifted if you are strong enough to hold it, or one arm can be lifted.

Teaching focus

- Go slowly so that the student can explore their limit and go at their own pace.

- Allow the student to modify the pose for their own ability and limitations.

- Provide encouragement within safe limits.

- Allow the student to stop at any time if they are not feeling safe.

Parkinson's/MS note: This is a little tricky for students with Parkinson's who are very stiff, but MS students will probably find it easier.

◼ Seated Warrior Pose 2

Use this pose for those unable to sustain balance in a standing position.

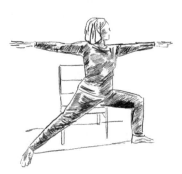

Instruction

1. Check the stability of the chair.

2. Sit up on the 'sit' bones near to the front edge of the chair seat, knees wide. Open the left knee, even wider, leg bent and angled out to the side, as far as the hip will allow. In order to do this, you may need to steady yourself using your arms for stability.

3. Slide the right leg straight and plant the foot firmly on the floor, hold the floor with the outside edge of the foot.

4. Once the legs are in position, core muscles can be engaged for strength.

5. Lift the arms to shoulder height, palms down; release the shoulders and lengthen the back of the neck.

6. With the head upright and neck long, look along the line of the arm and hand to complete the posture.

7. Return by lowering the arms to hold the chair and bring the legs back to parallel.

Teaching focus

- Engage core muscles.

- Release shoulder tension and offer other arm positions. Palms together in front of the chest, for example, or releasing the shoulders down and out, so that there is more softness in the trapezius.

- Stay connected to the floor – this encourages sure-footedness, anchoring into the ground.

- Check the knee and foot alignment – don't let the knees rotate inwards.

- With the chest open, practise full breathing.

- Strength, stability, courage and balance.

- Offer hands-on guidance for alignment and to areas that hold tension.

◼ Chair twisting postures

This is useful for those who cannot stand for an extended time, or who are unable to balance well enough, or if there is incidence of low blood pressure.

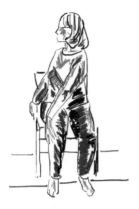 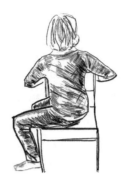

Instruction

Version 1:

1. Sit towards the front of the chair to give room for the turn.

2. Sit up onto the 'sit' bones and bring the spine upright, rather than a slumped back position.

3. Breathe in.

4. Take the left arm across the body, left hand to right knee. Exhaling, turn to the right, coordinating the breath with the movement.

5. Move the right hand around towards the back of the chair. Find a comfortable place for the hand and arm; this will depend on the type of chair.

Version 2: An option that gives more stretch is to sit sideways on the chair so that the chair back is to the side of the body.

1. Turn toward the back of the chair and hold it, using it to aid the turn. Keep the spine long.

2. Exhale and ease further into the turn.

Version 3: Use a block to aid the upper back and shoulder positioning.

1. Hold a firm block widthways out, at shoulder height.

2. Draw the shoulders down and back and let the little fingers engage firmly.

3. Turn to the right, and then to the left.

Teaching focus

In both standing and sitting versions of the twisting postures it is helpful to offer hands-on support, encouraging the shoulders to open and move down and back. This should be a light touch, as once the direction is given, the student will often very readily respond, and can manage further movement.

- Hands-on guidance can be helpful when there is a tendency for round shoulders or pulling away from the upright posture we want to encourage.

- Breathing up the spine in a spiral action. Feel that this is bringing prana into the spinal column.

- Lengthening both at the tail and crown – imagine creating spaces between the vertebrae.

- Good positioning of the shoulders to aid pectoral stretch acts as an antidote to round-shoulderedness.

- Root the tailbone down to the ground. Focus on Muladhara chakra.

- Breathe, and, in micro-movements on the exhale breath, increase the twist.

- Watch for the student tipping over to accommodate the back of the chair. Assist them in finding an arm position that does not pull the spine or shoulders out of alignment.

Parkinson's note: People with Parkinson's may develop a lopsidedness that often shows up in these twisting postures as a droop in one shoulder. Hands-on adjustment can bring awareness to this and promotes balanced working.

◼ Chair variation of Belly Twist Pose (Jathara Parivartanasana)

Instruction

1. Sit to the side of the chair with knees together, engage the pelvic floor and abdominals, sit up on the 'sit' bones, grow tall.

2. With arms stretched in front and palms together, turn away from the back of the chair as you open one arm out to the side.

3. Stay connected into the 'sit' bones, squeeze the knees together and feel that the breastbone turns. Let your arm open out but do not over-stretch.

Teaching focus

- Let the student lightly touch the breastbone with their fingertips, to focus on the centre of the turn. This will help resist the temptation to overdo it in the shoulder.

Note: The chair version is less effective and a little harder as students do not have the support of a flat surface to support the spine.

◼ Drawing a circle, chair version

You can add a further exploration of shoulder mobility by moving into 'Drawing a Circle', to encourage a full rotation at the shoulder.

Instruction

1. Sit on the chair to the side, to give free movement of the arm.

2. Hold the arms forwards at shoulder height with the palms together – imagine that you are going to draw a circle with your outer arm.

3. Breathing in, take the arm up above your head and around and down behind you as you breathe out, and then across the front hip and back to the start.

4. Imagine the trace of your fingers – draw a circle of light.

5. Repeat three times and then try circling in the other direction, before repeating the whole thing on the other side.

Teaching focus

- Explore the range of movement that the student can easily access.

- Check that the body is kept steady, and only the upper back turns.

- Do not force the hand to the floor; rather, allow the stretch and incremental progress.

This movement can help with a frozen shoulder, but may be limited if it is in an acute state.

■ Bound Angle Pose (or Cobbler Pose) (Baddha Konasana), with chair

You will need a block for this.

Instruction

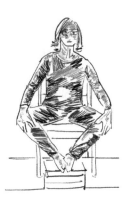

1. Sit towards the front of the chair and put your feet together on the block.

2. Let your knees drop apart, so that the soles of your feet come together.

3. Practise bringing your knees together and then letting them drop apart, creating a stretch in the adductors.

4. With the knees as wide apart as you can open them comfortably, take your arms back to hold the back of the chair.

5. Arch your spine back and breathe in.

6. Hold for three breaths.

7. Sit upright and bring the knees back together.

Teaching focus

- Opening the hip joints.

- Swadhistana chakra.

■ Chair Pose (Utkanasana), with a chair

Instruction

1. Sit on the 'sit' bones, knees together (feet can be on a block), hands in prayer position. Exhale and engage the pelvic floor – Mula Bhanda.

2. Draw in the abdominals and squeeze the knees together and connect your feet to the floor.

3. Hollow the spine and lean forward slightly, as if you are going to rise from the chair.

4. Lift your arms up, if you are able.

5. Breathe deeply for four breaths.

6. Lower your arms and return to a resting position.

■ Transferring: getting up and down out of a chair

This is something that we all need to work on as we get older, but needs to be practised so that we can build strength. This can usefully follow on from the semi-squat asanas.

Instruction

1. Sit on a chair. Practise using the pelvic floor and abdominal muscles. (This is emphasised throughout the book in almost all of the practices as it is an essential factor in stability, mobility and back care.)

2. Keep your feet parallel, and feel them on the floor. Press them into the floor, breathe out and engage the core.

3. Lean forward, keeping the natural curve in the spine, and, guiding the knees over the toes, reach the arms forward.

4. Follow the movement through by lifting off the chair just a few inches, and hold.

5. Try to sit down slowly and control the action. The chair *is* still there!

6. Practise this often.

Parkinson's/MS note: Initiating movements such as this can be a challenge. Often a signal to prepare and then move can make a huge difference. Simply counting helps to give the signal – for example, 'Engage the pelvic floor muscles, press the feet into the floor, 1, 2, 3, and lift.'

■ Leg lifts and chair bicycles

Instruction

1. Sit up tall, towards the front of the chair, and engage the core, bring your elbows in and lean back slightly, cross your hands over your heart. Try to do this without holding the chair, unless you have to.

2. Let your legs come forward a little and pick up your heels, toes on the ground.

3. Keeping the legs firm, lift one leg a foot or so off the floor. Maintain the angle of the knee – the movement should be in the hip and thigh.

4. Repeat four times on each side.

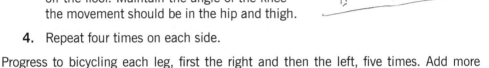

Progress to bicycling each leg, first the right and then the left, five times. Add more repetitions as you get stronger. Lying cycling exercises are on pages 92–93.

■ Chair balance

Instruction

1. Sit upright on your 'sit' bones, in the middle of the chair, and hold the seat with your hands.

2. Engage the core muscles and lean back.

3. Press your heels into the floor as if you are trying to pick your toes up.

4. Hold your lower leg in that position, while trying to maintain parallel knees, and lift one foot off the floor. It does not have to come up very far.

5. Do one at a time first of all, and then try lifting both.

6. When you get stronger, progress to extending your arms out to the sides, and hold.

7. Try different hand positions – palms together and then lifting them up, or raising arms parallel.

CHAIR-SUPPORTED STANDING POSTURES

■ Chair-supported Dancer Pose

This gives attention to the back-bending aspect of the balance and the length and openness through the front of the body from the knee up to the shoulders, but without the difficulty of the leg-back action.

Instruction

1. Place a chair with the back at the right-hand side for holding. You may need to put a block or cushion on the chair seat to get it at the right height – it should be easy to place a bent knee on the chair seat.

2. Hold the back of the chair with the right hand and place the right knee on the seat.

3. Extend the left arm up and move the hips forward, creating a mild back arch. Breathe in and stretch up.

4. Look up, moving the head slowly.

5. Lower the arm down, and repeat the stretching action three times. Relax and bring your knee off the seat.

6. Repeat with the left knee on the seat (moving to the other side of the chair is the easiest way).

Progress the stretch by lifting the heel of the standing foot to be on your toes, as you stretch up.

Teaching focus

- Keep the gaze ahead.
- Make sure that the chair is the right height.
- Hold the student steady at the hips if they are feeling wobbly.
- Give permission to opt out.

▇ Chair-supported Tree Pose

Instruction

1. Place the chair on the mat.
2. Stand next to the chair and lift one foot up onto the seat.
3. Either hold the back of the chair with one hand or bring both hands together, in prayer position.
4. Lift both hands or the free hand.

Teaching focus

- Growing roots.
- Level the pelvis.
- Toning the abdominal muscles to create a strong trunk.
- Breathe steadily.
- Stay focused.
- Affirmations: 'I am balanced and calm', 'Rooted in the earth, I grow to the light'.

◼ Standing chair-supported Warrior Pose 2

This follows on well from the chair-supported Tree Pose.

Instruction

1. Place the chair on the mat, or it could be placed side on to the wall.

2. Stand about 2 feet (40 cm) away from the chair, with the back of the chair to your right side. Keeping yourself steady with your hand on the chair, lift the right foot up onto the seat.

3. Turn the toes in of the left foot (on the floor).

4. Open your hips and bring your spine upright.

5. Let go of the chair back and lift both arms to shoulder height. Alternatively, keep hold of the chair back/wall.

6. Take care to come out of the posture step by step, remaining steady by holding the chair back, bringing the foot back to the floor.

Teaching focus

*   Strength and stability. Take this idea through from strength in the body to determination, achieving goals and mental strength.

◼ Chair- and wall-supported twist

The chair should be side-long against the wall.

Instruction

1. Stand facing the chair seat.

2. Lift the leg nearest the wall up onto the seat; your hip can be on the wall. Root the other foot firmly onto the floor.

3. Turn your shoulders and face the wall.

4. Place your hands on the wall and turn your body into the wall.

5. Return the foot to the floor and repeat on the other side.

Teaching focus

*   Keep the spine upright and bring a sense of enjoyment as the wall assists this twist.

*   Breathe along the spine.

*   Feel uplifted.

*   Focus on the toning of the spinal muscles and freeing up the spinal joints.

■ Chair-supported Cat Pose

This is a useful way to offer this posture. Blocks might be needed to adjust the height. Ideally, the spine should be level, but even with a slight angle, the spinal movement can be worked.

Instruction

1. With the chair seat facing you, lean forward and place your hands on the seat. Use blocks to provide height, if necessary. Shorter people might find it easier to put their elbows on the chair seat.

2. The feet should be parallel, or they could be wider, to bring the spine level.

3. Tilt the pelvis down and lift the tailbone as you breathe in and move your shoulder blades down your back.

4. Contract the pelvic floor and engage the abdominal muscles as you arch the back up as you breathe out.

5. Continue coordinating the movement and the breathing, allowing the spine to flex and extend.

Teaching focus

- Check the shoulder action – the shoulder blades should be sliding down the back to enable a good extension of the upper back.

- Visualise space through the spinal column.

From this position you can progress to some of the strengthening variations:

- Extend and curl: Stabilising on three points, without collapsing or dropping one hip, engage the abdominal muscles and pelvic floor muscles, lift and extend one leg, pushing the heel away. Stay steady throughout the move; try to keep the hips level. Keep everything as stable as possible on the return journey. Draw the leg right through and curl the nose towards the knee – this gives a natural balance to the action. Repeat using the other leg.

- Arm strengthening: Transfer the weight of the body forward so that the hands, arms and shoulders bear more, and then ease back. This enables the student to get used to taking weight onto the hands, and will help when transferring from lying to sitting to standing.

- Mini balance: Using the same position, lift the right arm out to the side, and lift the opposite leg away and back, so that there is balance on a diagonal basis.

- Knee circles: Stabilise over three points and lift one bent knee out to the side, lift the knee up, out and around, moving the hip joint. Repeat on the other leg.

■ Chair-supported Plank to Cobra Pose

Before offering this posture, check that your students have the strength and balance to do this. Some people with MS would find this hard because of balance issues and numbness in hands and feet. Offer the seated back bend as an alternative.

You will need a secure chair that is heavy enough to bear weight. Place the chair against the wall on the mat to prevent slipping.

Instruction

1. Stand 2 feet or so (40 cm) away from the chair. Bend forward and place your hands on the seat.

2. Tread your heels down into the floor, stretching your hamstrings.

3. Plank Pose: Take your weight onto your hands and bring your hips down, while keeping your legs as straight as possible, to get the whole body in a long line, from head to toe.

4. Cobra Pose: Lift the breastbone forwards, creating a back bend, and keep the shoulder blades moving down the back.

5. Come out of the pose by bringing your body upright, and step forward.

Teaching focus

- Check for safe practice.

- Building strength and confidence.

- Stretches hamstrings.

- Check that this movement is within the capabilities of the student.

■ Gate Pose from the chair

Instruction

1. Sit towards the front of the chair, feet parallel.

2. Take the right leg out to the side.

3. Place your right hand on the leg, and begin to slide it down the leg.

4. Lift your left arm up and over to create a crescent moon shape.

5. Hold and breathe into the stretch.

6. Keep the shoulders aligned over one another, so as not to twist forwards.

7. Return, bringing your right arm down and your spine upright.

8. Repeat on the other side.

Teaching focus

- Alignment.

- Staying rooted in the 'sit' bones.

- Visualise the space between your knee, ribs and fingertips.
- Visualise the crescent moon shape – imagine holding a moon in your arms.
- Align the head and neck.

■ Downward-facing Dog Pose, seated version

Instruction

1. Pull the chair close up to the wall, and sit on the chair with the wall in front of you, feet parallel.
2. Reach out and up, and place your hands on the wall a little wider apart than your shoulders.
3. Press against the wall and lean in. Create an extension in your spine and stretch through the shoulders.
4. Walk your hands higher.
5. Stay at the end of your range and breathe. Hold for five breaths.
6. Walk your hands back down and soften your shoulders.

■ Simple seated 'Sun' flow

Throughout this sequence, encourage coordinated breathing and a flowing movement. Focus on the practice being fun rather than precise.

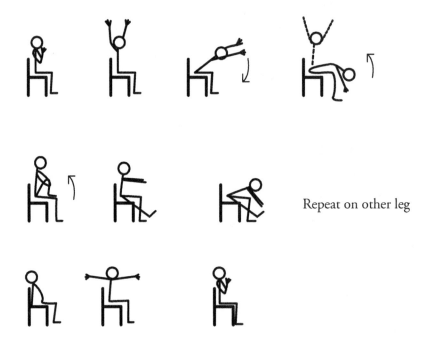

Repeat on other leg

Instruction

1. Sit up on the 'sit' bones, with feet parallel and arms relaxed and down by your sides.

2. Bring the palms together in front of your chest. Namaste. Exhale.

3. Inhale and part your hands, taking your arms up above in 'salutation'.

4. Exhale and hinge from the hips and bend forwards; keep your spine and arms in a long line.

5. Bring your hands to the floor and drop your head down. Take a couple of easy breaths.

6. Inhale and lift your spine up in a relaxed way, to sit up.

7. Draw your right knee in, exhaling. Hold the knee with both hands.

8. Inhale and stretch your right leg out straight, sliding the foot along the floor.

9. Exhale and bend over the straight leg, sliding your hands down along the leg. Keep lengthening your spine.

10. Lift your arms up as you lift out of the bend.

11. Sweep your arms around to hold the back or sides of the chair.

12. Arch the back, lifting the breastbone.

13. Exhale and hug the left knee in.

14. Inhale and stretch your left leg out straight, sliding the foot along the floor.

15. Exhale and bend over the straight leg, sliding your hands down along the leg. Keep lengthening your spine.

16. Lift your arms up as you lift out of the bend, inhaling.

17. Exhale and bring your hands to hold the chair at the back corners, and bring the breastbone forwards into a seated back arch as you inhale.

18. Hold for a breath.

19. On an inhale breath, sweep your arms out to the sides and lift them above the head, palms together.

20. Bring the hands back to the chest. Namaste.

21. Repeat four times.

Teaching focus

- Breath coordination and keeping the flow.
- Heart energy, Anahata.
- It doesn't matter how 'raggedy' the movement is – let there be joy in the accomplishment.
- You may be able to introduce other points for awareness as the student becomes more experienced.

Flow sequences

Postures that work in a sequence of flowing movements are a useful, beneficial and enjoyable part of therapeutic yoga practice. They:

- improve coordination

- exercise the muscles of the heart

- improve breathing

- improve circulation

- improve joint mobility

- aid memory.

Traditional flow sequences are the Sun salutation, Moon salutation series and those familiar to Ashtanga yoga practitioners.

Difficulty in sequencing, joint stiffness, cramps, fear, weakness and numbness may all hinder the student in getting to grips with the traditional flow sequences as we know them. However, most students love to try them, which in itself is empowering. Flow sequences may be contraindicated where students have painful swollen joints, for example; other contraindications should be evaluated before attempting the flow practices.

Here are some ideas for flow sequences that can be used with Parkinson's and MS groups. I have included some seated sequences and some floor work. I suggest the following adaptations and teaching the sequence in steps for a gradual build-up. Use some of the individual postures such as Cat, Dog, extended Child, Swan and Cobra, to build awareness of how the postures can connect together and build strength.

■ Simple seated 'Sun' flow

Throughout this sequence, encourage coordinated breathing and flowing movement. Focus on the practice being fun rather than precise.

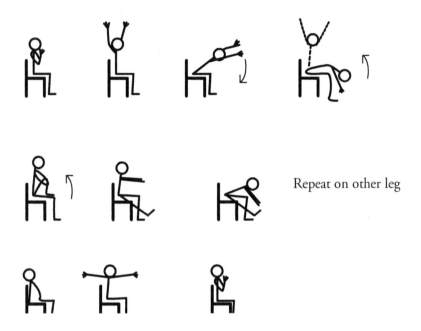

Repeat on other leg

Instruction

1. Sit up on the 'sit' bones, with feet parallel and arms relaxed and down by your sides.

2. Bring the palms together in front of your chest. Namaste. Exhale.

3. Inhale and part your hands, taking your arms up above in 'salutation'.

4. Exhale and hinge from the hips and bend forwards; keep your spine and arms in a long line.

5. Bring your hands to the floor and drop your head down. Take a couple of easy breaths.

6. Inhale and lift your spine up in a relaxed way, to sit up.

7. Draw your right knee in, exhaling. Hold the knee with both hands.

8. Inhale and stretch your right leg out straight, sliding the foot along the floor.

9. Exhale and bend over the straight leg, sliding your hands down along the leg. Keep lengthening your spine.

10. Lift your arms up as you lift out of the bend.

11. Sweep your arms around to hold the back or sides of the chair.

12. Arch the back, lifting the breastbone.

13. Exhale and hug the left knee in.

14. Inhale and stretch your left leg out straight, sliding the foot along the floor.

15. Exhale and bend over the straight leg, sliding your hands down along the leg. Keep lengthening your spine.

16. Lift your arms up as you lift out of the bend, inhaling.

17. Exhale and bring your hands to hold the chair at the back corners, and bring the breastbone forwards into a seated back arch as you inhale.

18. Hold for a breath.

19. On an inhale breath, sweep your arms out to the sides and lift them above the head, palms together.

20. Bring the hands back to the chest. Namaste.

Build up the number of repeats according to your ability and energy.

Teaching focus

- Breath coordination and keeping the flow.
- Heart energy, Anahata.
- It doesn't matter how 'raggedy' the movement – let there be joy in the accomplishment whatever the level.
- You may be able to introduce other points for awareness as the student becomes more experienced.

■ Warrior flow

Use a chair for support, although this may not be needed in some cases.

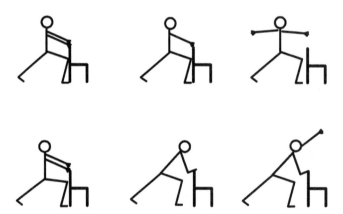

Instruction

1. Stand facing the back of the chair, feet together in parallel. Step back with the right foot, and angle the left foot, so that feet are ready for Warrior Pose. The front knee is bent, hands lightly touching the back of the chair.

2. Lift the right arm, and as you lower it, lift the left arm. Making a scissor-type movement with the arms. Coordinate this with breathing (this can be paced to work with the student's need). Repeat six times.

3. As you lift the right arm, continue taking it up and around until it is at shoulder height in the position we know as Warrior Pose 2, at the same time allowing the body to turn to the side, arms outstretched. The left hand can stay on the back of the chair for support, if needed.

4. Hold for a breath (the number of breaths can increase as strength improves).

5. Lower the right arm down and bring it back to the chair back. Turn the hips to face the chair back.

6. Bend both elbows out to the sides and lean in to create a long diagonal line, from foot to crown.

7. Lift one arm along the same line; lift both if there is strength and balance.

8. Repeat with the other leg forward.

Teaching focus

- Create a strong core.

- Coordination of breath and movement.

- Bring attention into the body and direct an enquiry: Where do we feel strong? Which parts do not work as well as we would like?

- Keep bringing awareness into the feet.

- Accept what is.

■ Cat–Dog–Swan flow

This short sequence can serve as a preliminary for the kneeling Sun Salutation.

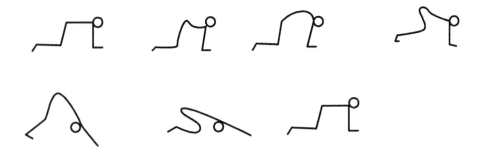

Instruction

1. Kneeling on the mat in Cat Pose (see page 51), check your alignment.

2. Inhale and lift the tailbone, hollow the spine. Exhale and arch the spine (Cat/Cow Pose, see page 51). Repeat four times.

3. Lift the knees, tread the heels back into the floor and then lower both heels. Breathe steadily through this.

4. Shift the weight back and lengthen the spine into Downward-facing Dog Pose (see page 106).

5. Bend the knees and lower them back to the ground.

6. Sit back onto the heels as far as possible, and stretch the arms forwards, along the mat.

7. Move back to the starting Cat Pose and repeat the Cat/Cow movements. (The whole thing can be repeated according to the student's stamina.)

8. Rest in semi-supine with curled-up legs afterwards.

Teaching focus

*   The hips, knees and spine are the focal areas, and may also be problem areas. Allow the students to find their own level of moving – a 'do what you can do today' approach.

*   Foster acceptance.

*   Use the words: grace, fun, flow.

*   Stop whenever you like, enabling self-awareness and taking out any competitive element.

■ Upward-facing and Downward-facing Dog Pose with a chair

Place a chair with its back to the wall. This makes sure that the student is safe.

Instruction

1. Step back a little way, legs hip-width apart, and bend to grip the chair seat at each side.

2. Lean the hips into the chair, stretch the hamstrings first, but let the heels come up if the legs are tight.

3. Press your hands into the chair, arms straight, and lift the spine up, chest forwards, into Cobra Pose (see pages 62–63).

4. Bend at the hips and push the tailbone back, lengthening the spine. Keep the legs straight if possible, at the same time stretch through the shoulders.

5. Repeat from the beginning, four times.

Teaching focus

- Counteracts round shoulders and a rounding spine.
- Stretches the hamstrings.
- Flexibility of the spine.

■ Kneeling Sun Salutation

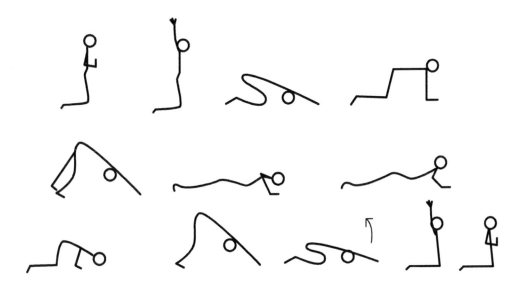

This requires some strength and mobility, so will not suit everyone. It can be edited and shortened to allow students to work at their own level. It is suitable for students who may have problems standing or with their balance, but will help to build strength if practised in stages.

Instruction

1. Start in an upright kneeling position, towards the front of the mat.
2. Inhale and raise your arms up above your head in Salutation Pose.
3. Exhale and bend forwards, sitting back into your heals and stretching your arms along the mat in Swan Pose (see page 109).
4. Inhale and move onto 'all fours', into Cat Pose (see page 51).
5. Move the spine as you would in Cat/Cow Pose (see page 51).
6. Exhale and lift your knees, treading back into Downward-facing Dog Pose (see page 106). Inhale and bring the knees back to the floor.
7. Exhale and stretch your arms forward along the mat and slide your body forward to lie flat, face down. You can move straight to Cat Pose if you are not strong enough to move through the Cobra part of the sequence.

8. Breathe normally. (Rest here if needed.)

9. Place your hands under the shoulders in readiness.

10. Exhale and engage the core muscles before lifting the head and chest to move into a modified Cobra. Inhale.

11. Exhale as you move your hands down to waist level, press into the floor, and lift your hips to return to Cat Pose.

12. Exhale and lift your knees, treading back into Downward-facing Dog Pose. Inhale and bring the knees back to the floor.

13. Extend your arms along the mat into Swan Pose (see page 109), with the exhale breath.

14. Inhale and lift your arms and spine to stand on your knees, arms stretched up in Salutation Pose.

15. Exhale and lower your arms and bring hands into Namaste, to complete the sequence.

Teaching focus

- Break the sequence down and teach it in parts, building up over time to the full sequence.

- Even in this kneeling version, students will need enough strength to support their body through the Cobra section. Prepare with stamina-building postures in the weeks running up to it.

- Allow the student to do what they can and to miss parts that are too difficult.

- Give general rules for breathing such as 'breathe in as you open out and breathe out as you bend and fold', so that if they get lost they can pick up the flow.

- Focus on mobility, energy flow and enjoyment in the movement rather than achieving a perfect flow.

- Repeats can be added as the students gain strength, confidence and stamina.

Breathing

In yoga we use the word Pranayama, often in direct reference to the breath, and yet the word prana is about life force, the very essence of our being alive. When we talk about disruption in the flow of prana, we are talking about the ill health of the functions of the body. Breathing is divided into four parts: inhaling (puraka), breath retention (antar kumbhaka), exhaling (recaka) and being empty (bahya kumbhaka).

There are numerous methodologies and techniques practising Pranayama. The ultimate aim is to enhance the life force, and to improve the physical function of breathing; because of the link with the nervous system, we can soothe the mind and restore balance.

When lungs work more efficiently, we take in more energy – that is, oxygen – and we feel more vital and alive. The alveoli can become clogged and congested, and so as we improve our breathing, and this congestion clears, the lung tissue becomes more elastic, and with better lung function, health improves. In people with MS and Parkinson's, breathing well will mean fewer infections and a more robust constitution. When we take in more oxygen, the heart and circulation benefit. The heart rate changes with different breathing patterns, some linked with boosting energy and others with calming. The intercostal muscles in the chest and back begin to work better, giving us greater control over our breathing.

Breathing helps to bring about a state of relaxation – as we slow it down, we calm the nervous system, and the movement of the breath affects the vagus nerve. It is vital as preparation for relaxation. If there is fear, upset or distress, the diaphragm often becomes tight, and in spasm, breathing can bring about a release, which might be emotional as well as physical.

In Parkinson's there is a tendency towards greater anxiety. This will worsen physical symptoms. In MS and Parkinson's, low-energy states and tiredness are common, and an improvement in breathing will make positive changes to energy levels with practice.

So, the benefits of breathing are as follows:

- improves lung capacity

- improves elasticity of the lung tissue

- benefits the heart muscle

- improves circulation

- exercises the muscles of the chest and upper back

- releases the diaphragm

- helps to relax body and mind

- better oxygen exchange makes more energy available, therefore we feel less tired.

People with MS or Parkinson's may have had no experience of yoga or of healthy breathing practices before coming to a special yoga class or one-to-one session. This will mean starting with the basics.

Posture will make a huge difference to the ability to breathe well. A rounded upper spine, rigid pectoral muscles and tight sternocleidomastoid will mean that the breathing apparatus cannot function optimally.

Pranayama has three main effects: brmhana, langhana and samana.

- Brmhana is the effect where more energy is produced. This comes from putting the focus on inhalation and then on the hold after inhalation. At the conclusion of a brmhana practice, the practitioner feels an expansion of the chest area (and the lungs), and a good sensation of balanced energy will follow.

- Langhana is a calming and interiorising effect, mainly because the focus is on exhalation and on the hold after exhalation. The lungs are empty and langhana can produce a calming effect, the mind easily focusing in the abdominal area.

- Samana is a balanced harmonising effect resulting from a combination of brmhana and langhana. The mind becomes focused.

These different effects can be introduced into the class where and when it is appropriate, bearing in mind that a common symptom of Parkinson's is low blood pressure, and practices will need to be chosen with this in mind.

The breathing practices detailed here are not strictly classical Pranayama; they are designed to improve the function of breathing. Unless otherwise stated, breathing should always be through the nose. This warms the air, filters out dust and dirt, and prepares the air for entry into the body. Many improvements in health can be made by nose breathing.

■ Begin with awareness

From a seated position, allow time for the students to explore how they are breathing in everyday life. Do they ever notice that they are short of breath? Do they breathe slowly or quickly? Does their breathing pattern change alongside other symptoms or medication? Are there times when they feel they 'don't breathe'? Do they experience panic or fear? It is helpful to open up this kind of discussion before starting to teach breathing practices.

Invite the group to breathe normally, and notice where they are breathing, how and where the body moves. Which part of the breath is easier – breathing out or breathing in? Is it long, smooth, easy or rushed and grasped? These observations lead to an understanding of the mental activity directing the breath. The breath is an indicator.

If the student is able to come to the floor, semi-supine position is an excellent position to bring awareness to the breath. Encourage the group to place their hands on the belly, on the chest or along their sides to find where the movement of breathing happens.

■ Abdominal breathing

For these particular groups who have Parkinson's or MS, the seated position is the best choice to begin, sitting not too far back in the chair so that the student can feel into the back of the body and possibly even reach their hands around to touch it lightly.

Instruction

1. Place your fingertips so that they just meet above the navel, empty the lungs, focus on directing air into the diaphragm, and allow a gentle movement to move the hands apart – 'breathe into your hands'.

2. Take care that you don't force the abdomen out; it should be a natural relaxed way of breathing. Moving hands to touch the front, sides and back can help increase awareness of the breath moving around the whole circumference.

■ Thoracic breathing

Instruction

1. Hook your thumbs under your armpits, palms down.

2. Direct the breath into the middle of the chest. Focus on the ribcage lifting up and out.

3. Allow the fingers to move away from each other, also touching the front, sides and back, but around the rib circumference.

■ Clavicular breathing

Instruction

1. Place your fingertips just under the collarbone. Fill the bottom and middle, and continue until you feel a little movement under the collarbone; the shoulders will lift a little.

There are many other ways that we can become aware of breath in that these separate compartments and this awareness can be carried through the asana and meditation practices.

■ Individual observation

It is useful to spend time observing the student breathing. A semi-supine position is good to start, or standing, if the student is able.

Get the student to breathe fully, and observe carefully where there is freedom of movement. Check:

- the abdomen

- action in the ribcage

- movement in the clavicular area

- if there is any straining around the throat

- the quality of the breath – is there any sense of grasping the breath, or is there a smooth flow?

Bring the student's awareness to any areas of limitation, ask what they notice about this and how it feels to them. Use conscious awareness to bring energy and breath into any 'frozen' areas. Ask permission to touch, and place a hand lightly on the area to aid awareness and encourage the muscles that might be holding tight to release. I find that using images, colour and focus allow changes to happen – a simple instruction to soften an area or 'change the colour' will instigate change. Continue to work in this way until the breath begins to free up, and becomes easier, smooth and relaxed.

This kind of breath awareness work can be brought into a small group (four would be workable), but does present a challenge in offering the kind of guidance that will make a difference for each individual. Instruction would have to be general.

BREATHING PRACTICES

■ Full yoga breath (Mahat Pranayama)
This is often termed as the 'three-part breath'.

Instruction

1. Putting all three experiences together, with one hand on the abdomen and the other on the upper part of the chest, breathe slowly, filling from the bottom to the top, and emptying from the top to the bottom.

The relaxing effect of this full 'yoga' breath is experienced in semi-supine position, and, taught in this position, gives the student the means to soothe and calm themselves. This beneficial calming property of breathing practice will enable the student to practise at home, when they are feeling anxious or agitated, or in preparation for sleep. Use different methods over time so that the student stays engaged with the idea of breath improvement. Arm movement coordination can assist the student to understand and feel the action of the breathing.

■ Arm–breath coordination in three-part breathing
Both of these can be done sitting, standing or supine.

Instruction

1. Begin very simply, with arms relaxed down by the sides of the body. Breathe out. Begin to breathe in and turn the palms out, turn the palms back again on the exhale breath, breathing down into the abdomen with this movement. Repeat a few times and then let the arm movement increase, as the breath comes higher into the chest, first to shoulder height, and finally a full breath, with arms fully extended.

2. Begin with the arms down by the sides and empty the lungs. Breathe into the abdomen and lift the arms to shoulder height, palms down. Turn the palms to face in and continue to inhale as you open the arms out. Continue the inhale

breath right up into the clavicle, as you lift your arms above your head. Sweep the arms forward and down on the exhale breath.

Many simple movements can support the function of breathing. Lifting the arms above on an in-breath and lowering on an out-breath will help the upper back, ribcage and chest to move. Likewise, with palms together and arms outstretched at shoulder height, and then opening them on an inhale breath and closing them on an exhale breath can bring the widthways movements into focus. These gentle approaches to breathwork can be done a little at a time, and in this way are not contraindicated for blood pressure problems unless they are done standing up, when dizziness may occur if there is low blood pressure.

◼ Bronchial problems and asthma

People with Parkinson's and MS may also have bronchial conditions, so these small practices can help to support them in this aspect of their health. The following practices are useful for enabling the muscles used in breathing to work well.

◼ Incremental/stepped breathing

Measured incremental exhale breath (krama) engages the intercostal muscles and diaphragm, and improves elasticity of the tissue.

Instruction

1. Sit or stand, and take a full inhale breath, through the nose.

2. Breathe out in short puffs through the mouth, making a quiet 'peh' sound as you do it. Don't suck air in; continue to 'puff' air out until you have none left, and the lungs are very empty. Or you could count ten puffs and then let the rest of the air out smoothly. Repeat three or four times.

Progress can be made by counting the 'puffs', and seeing if the practice can be extended by counting up to a higher number.

Teaching focus

*   Check the technique – there should be no inhale breath between the 'steps'.

*   Imagine the lung tissue and muscles as stretchy and elastic.

*   Feel in control of the process.

The technique can be done in reverse, breathing in the air in measured 'sips' through the mouth, and exhaling through the nose.

Enhancing the technique

*   Other ways to enhance the technique can be by beginning with a given count, say six, and raising the arms a little on each count until they are fully lifted on the final count; this will encourage the lift of the ribs. Over the weeks this can be extended by increasing the count.

*   Visual imaging can also help. I use the analogy of taking the breaths up the steps and down the lift.

Caution: These methods are meant to be preventative, and will not necessarily be of help during an asthmatic 'attack'.

■ Slow breathing

It has been shown that slow breathing has the effect of calming the vagus nerves and switching off the stress response. A number of techniques can be practised to bring the breathing rate down to five or six breaths per minute. Balanced ratio breathing is good practice for this, as well as improving control and working the diaphragm.

Instruction

1. Start very slowly and avoid holding on the exhale or inhale breath.

2. Use the idea of the three-part breath and divide the inhale; breathe into bottom, middle and top with an even count for each, starting with four.

3. Exhale and begin the inhale into the bottom section for a count of four, then the middle section for a count of four, and then the upper part for four. Exhale for a count of 12.

4. Progress the practice breathing into the three sections for 5 and out to 15, and so on, a count of five in each part progressing to a greater number with time. Breathing out should last the same amount of time as the inhale. Over time the rate of breathing can be slow and comfortable. After each round of breathing (say four breaths), rest.

Teaching focus

- Let the students work at a speed that is comfortable for them.
- Encourage home practice.

If anyone is 'short' of breath, let them work at their own pace and rest where necessary. Breathing practices sometimes provoke coughing. Coughing is the body's way of clearing the lungs – make it okay for people to cough in class.

■ Encourage a long exhale

This is useful for asthmatics who need to practise when they are not in an asthmatic spasm, to feel confident that they have the ability to breathe out, and to be able to relax with it.

The ratio here is to extend the out-breath for three times the length of the in-breath. Inhaling for a count of four, exhaling for 12, and then slowing the whole process down by adding a number.

Instruction

1. Take the arms back a little, drawing the shoulder blades down to open the chest.

2. Take a full breath to a count of four; make sure that the whole of the lungs are filled at four.

3. Exhale for a count of 12.

4. Breathe in to five, out to 15, in to six, out to 18, and then in to five, out to 15, in to four, out to 12 – five breaths in all.

■ Awareness and muscle tone

This can be done sitting or standing, stretching the upper back.

Instruction

1. With hands clasped together under the chin, breathe in, and push gently upward, bringing the chin up, as the elbows are opened out.

2. Breathe out as you bring your hands and elbows down.

■ Expansion

This is designed to bring an awareness of expanding the chest and encouraging horizontal, vertical and side expansion.

Instruction

1. Horizontal expansion: Stretch the arms forward at shoulder height, palms together. Exhale first and then open the arms wide on the inhale breath. Close on the exhale breath. Repeat five times.

2. Vertical expansion: Begin with the arms down by the sides and lift them up on the inhale breath, lower on the exhale breath.

3. Side expansion: Inhaling, lean over to one side and draw the arm up with the elbow bent and the fist curled up into the armpit. Repeat three times on each side.

Teaching focus

•   Keep the mental focus to match the intention of the practice – that is, imagine the lungs/ribcage expanding.

•   Visualise the breath as a golden light bringing in energy.

•   Promoting the flow of prana.

•   Chest opening, lungs elastic and healthy.

■ Breathing 'into one lung'

This interesting practice is also an exercise in mental focus and awareness.

Instruction

1. Bring the fingertips to touch across the chest.

2. Focus your attention into the right lung.

3. Breathe in and imagine the air going only into the right lung. Imagine the left lung staying empty (like an empty balloon in the left side).

4. Do this three times, feeling the movement of your hand and how the fingers move apart.

5. Take a deep full breath, using the whole of the lungs.

6. Repeat with awareness in filling the left side, and leaving the right side empty.

7. End with full breathing, with the whole of the lungs expanding.

◼ Decongesting

Tapping and rubbing as you exhale can help to decongest the lungs. This is useful to practise if there is residue following a cold, for example.

Instruction

1. Breathe in fully and rub up and down over the lower part of the ribcage – front and sides are easy to get to, but help may be needed with the back part.

2. Breathe in fully, and, using the fists, gently hit the upper chest in a 'Tarzan' action. Again, help will be needed to get to the back.

3. Breathe in fully and exhale while tapping over the whole of the chest with the fingertips.

More forceful cleansing can happen with Chopping breath and the Ha breath. Care needs to be taken with balance and any back problems. Both of these can be done from a chair.

◼ Chopping breath

This is usually done from a standing legs-apart position, but a chair version can work just as well.

Instruction

1. Clasp your hands, stretch them up as high as possible as you inhale through the nose, and then bring them down forcefully on exhaling through the mouth, as if you are chopping wood.

2. Let the knees bend. Repeat four times. Coughing may occur after this.

Teaching focus

- It is helpful and safer to engage the core muscles to do this.
- Check for balance.
- Offer a chair if needed.
- Explain that coughing is a normal result of this practice.
- This is contraindicated if there are disc problems.

◼ Ha breath

This is a slightly gentler version of Chopping breath.

Instruction

1. Stand, feet apart. Raise your arms as high as possible, inhaling through the nose; drop the arms and the body forwards with the knees bent, exhaling through the mouth.

2. Hang over in a loose manner, with bent knees. This dropped position can be held for a short time to help the chest to drain. Again, there may be coughing.

◼ Helping the diaphragm to work

This is better used in a one-to-one situation with the teacher working hands-on, but it can be directed to a small group.

With the student lying in semi-supine, stand with your feet apart near to their feet so that you can easily place your hands on the sides of the ribcage (not the front). Instruct the student to inhale and then, as they exhale, gently press inwards as if you are helping the lungs to empty. Keep going until the end of the exhale breath, and instruct the student to breathe in naturally as you let go. The intake of air will expand the chest and work the diaphragm, giving a feeling of release.

When instructing a small group, the students should lie in the same position as described above, and place their own hands on the sides of their chest (although this is not always possible). They can then inhale and begin to squeeze inwards to facilitate the exhale breath. Please note that this is a gentle pressure, not a rib-cracking one. When they feel ready to breathe in again, they let go and breathe in freely.

◼ Coordination and awareness

In the following practices, coordinated movements are to enable the mind to focus on finding a match between the breath and body. These can be done from a standing or sitting position.

◼ Complete breath

Instruction

1. Start with arms down by your sides in comfortable Mountain Pose (Tadasana) (see page 78).

2. Exhale, begin to breathe in, and at the same time, lift the arms out and up. Aim to let the arms meet above the head, palms together, as the lungs are fully filled.

3. Begin the return journey as you breathe out, to let the arms come back to rest down by your sides as the lungs are empty. Take time and a few repeats to make adjustments to this practice. There is no hurry.

The whole practice should be calming.

Teaching focus

- Smooth breathing.

- Go just as far as the breath will allow.

- Go slowly.

- It may eventually be possible to rise onto the toes at the same time as the breath and arm movement begins, returning and lowering the heels.

■ 'Welcome' breath

Instruction

1. Begin standing or sitting with palms together in front of your heart. Take a few calm, smooth breaths and focus your attention in the heart centre.

2. Breathe out comfortably, and as you begin to inhale, move your arms forwards, opening outwards, feeling as if you are 'welcoming' the breath in.

3. Open your arms as wide as possible – feel that the chest is open and the heart is open.

4. Bring your arms back to the starting position, exhaling. Repeat five times and then wait quietly, with your attention focused in the heart.

Teaching focus

- Awareness of the heart chakra, Anahata, bringing in life and energy.

- Feel the openness of the chest, stretching into the pectoral area and then releasing.

- Are you willing to be open or not?

■ Breathing for relaxation and meditation

These techniques are designed to calm the mind; they engage mental faculty through image and sound.

■ White board

Instruction

1. Sit or stand. Imagine that you have in front of you a white board, and you hold in your hands black marker pens. Breathe out.

2. As you begin to breathe in, imagine drawing two parallel black lines up the white board. See them standing out, sharp and clear.

3. At the top of the breath, imagine you are holding two soft cloths, and on the exhale breath imagine that you are wiping away the lines, leaving the board clean and clear. The black lines represent your tensions and worries.

4. Draw them again as you breathe in, the black standing out against the white.

5. Wipe them away on the out-breath, as if you are wiping away your tensions and worries.

6. Take a third breath and repeat the process; deep black lines are wiped away on the exhale breath as a symbol of wiping away your worries and anxieties.

Colour breathing

Choose three colours to work with. The method is to imagine breathing in a colour, to visualise the colour filling the lungs, and then imagine breathing it out through the skin.

Instruction

1. Imagine a beautiful sapphire blue. Breathe in and imagine this colour filling your lungs – beautiful sapphire blue, breathing in the qualities of calm and peace.

2. As you breathe out, feel as if you are breathing out through every pore of your body, back as well as front; imagine the colour radiating out all around you. Repeat this three times, and then pause and imagine that you are sitting in a cloud of sapphire blue, the qualities of peace and calm surround you.

3. Let the colour fade.

4. Move on to the next colour.

Three colours is enough to work with at one time, as more begins to be confusing.

Give the students an option to opt out; if they don't 'get' it, many will not be able to visualise a colour, but may be able to imagine the qualities that are connected. Suggestions for colours are:

Red	strength and energy
Orange	courage and confidence
Yellow	clarity and upliftment
Green	sympathy and harmony
Blue	peace and calm
Indigo	absolute stillness
Violet	creativity and inspiration

Classic Pranayamas

These are good practices to develop concentration in preparation for meditation. Most students use them to feel calm and balance and to reduce anxiety.

■ Humming Bee Breath (Bhramari)

Instruction

1. Relax and practise a few rounds of full breathing.

2. Relax your jaw, with your lips gently closed.

3. Place your fingers on the flaps of your ears and press inwards gently, to 'close' the ears.

4. Inhale, and on the exhale breath make a deep steady humming sound continue for the length of the exhalation. Avoid having your teeth together.

5. Alternatively, without placing your fingers in your ears, move your tongue to the back of the mouth on the out-breath and make the sound 'ng', as in song; hold the sound as long as you have breath.

6. Breathe in deeply and repeat.

7. Keep going for a little time, and then spend some time in silence.

■ Alternate nostril breathing

Instruction

1. Bring your right hand to your face.

2. Place your thumb against your right nostril and another finger to the left.

3. Close your left nostril and breathe in through the right.

4. Close the right and breathe out through the left.

5. Breathe in through the left.

6. Close the left, and breathe out through the right.

7. This completes one round of breathing. Repeat four times.

■ Ujjayi breath

This Pranayama enhances chest breathing and amplifies the energy (prana) coming into the body. It brings a sense of strength and power, but with calm and steadiness. Breathing through the nostrils, the inhale breath is drawn through a half-closed glottis to make a sound both on the in- and out-breath. You will be able to hear this.

Parkinson's note: This technique may be difficult as laryngeal function and vocal muscles are weakened in some people with Parkinson's. According to Parkinson's UK, 95 per cent of people with Parkinson's have difficulty swallowing. Any beneficial effect of Ujjayi for these symptoms remains to be discovered.

■ Healing and energy focus

'Pranic healing' is yoga's healing methodology. There is no research as yet to ascertain whether it has any actual healing value, but we have used it here to promote positive thoughts, and to engage people with the idea that they are empowered to do something active for their health and wellbeing. These techniques were taught by my first yoga teacher, in the 1970s.

■ Pressing the prana

Instruction

1. Stand or sit. Bring your arms on to your chest with the fingers interlaced or hand softly held, palms in.

2. Breathe in and take your arms forwards away from the body, as if you are breathing into the space between your hands and your body; visualise your breath as if it is full of sparkling light.

3. Draw your arms in, to rest on your chest as you exhale – imagine that you are absorbing the prana into your chest. Repeat this three times.

4. Move your hands onto your head.

5. Breathe out, and then stretch the arms up above as you inhale, with the same idea of filling this space, between your arms and head.

6. On the exhale breath, 'press' the prana into the head and imagine that you are absorbing it. Repeat this three times.

Viewing this practice from the point of view of prana vayu, we are influencing both Udana and Vyana, at the same time stimulating the subtle energy in Anahata and Sahasrara.

■ Storing pranic energy

Instruction

1. From a comfortable seated position, visualise taking the prana in as you inhale. Feel that you are sending the energy to the solar plexus centre, as if you have a battery there, and you are recharging your battery with your breath. Hold your attention here for a short time, suspending the breath, and then breathe out. Repeat five times. This supports Manipura chakra and samana.

Once we have built our store of energy, we can envisage this as spreading throughout the body to nourish any part that feels in need or depleted.

■ Savitri Pranayama

Savitri Pranayama is a rhythmic breathing practice that has positive health benefits. The 2:1 rhythm is said to have various effects according to the length of the breath, which produces a different rhythm. Below is a summary of the different rhythms and their influences:

- 16:8 master breath (contains all others)
- 4:2 influences the glandular system

- 6:3 emotions
- 8:4 body, breath, cellular structures grounding
- 10:5 metabolism
- 12:6 mind clearing
- 14:7 stillness throughout
- 16:8 rejuvenation on all levels.

The 6:3 rhythm is a good starting place and will bring a sense of calm. This Pranayama can be done lying in Corpse Pose (Savasana) (see page 229), for a calming effect.

■ Cooling breaths

These two practices are the only ones where breathing in through the mouth is used. This contracts the blood vessels in the mouth, thereby affecting the whole face and head. These are useful if the student can master them, although for reasons stated before, the vocal apparatus and facial muscles may be weakened, so it may take time. Hissing sound breath (Sitkari) will be easier.

■ Hissing sound breath (Sitkari)

Instruction

1. Inhale through your mouth by placing your tongue behind your teeth and draw the air in, making a hissing sound; this has a cooling effect. When your lungs are filled, breathe out through the nose.

■ Crow's beak breath (Sitali)

Instruction

1. Extend the tongue out a little way, and curl the edges into a tube, and draw the breath in through this tube. At the end of the breath, draw the tongue in and exhale through the nose.

Note: Some people are genetically unable to perform this movement.

Relaxation and visualisation

Relaxation and the stress response

Many people think of yoga as being mainly physically focused practices, and even when yoga is used as a therapy, there is often a perception that we are looking for a posture to fix this or that. Here we present the relaxation practices as some of the most powerful tools in our therapeutic 'Yoga medicine bag'.

What is stress and how does it affect Parkinson's disease and multiple sclerosis?

When a person is subject to stressors, the brain makes a quick decision: 'Does this benefit or threaten me?' The strength of the response that follows depends on the answer to this question. This is a very individual thing. One person's stress is another's thrill (eustress); what one sees as a pressure, another will be excited by the challenge.

The 'fight or flight' mechanism springs into action whenever we feel threatened; it doesn't matter whether the threat is real or imagined, or whether it is in response to a physical danger or a perceived mental or emotional one – the effect is the same. The brain triggers chemical changes, which enable the body to respond to the danger. This is what happens:

- Cortisone is released – protecting us from an allergic reaction, for example, from dust.

- The thyroid speeds up the metabolism to allow fuel to burn faster and to release energy.

- Endorphins are released – these are natural painkillers, similar to morphine.

- The body shuts down the systems not needed to fight – these are the reproductive system, so sex hormones are reduced. The digestive tract shuts down as blood is diverted to the heart, lungs and muscles.

- Adrenaline is released into the system.

- Sugar is released, for a short-duration energy supply.

- Cholesterol is released from the liver to help transport long duration fuels to the muscles.

- The heartbeat races as the heart speeds up to supply the lungs and muscles with oxygen and fuel.

- Air supply is increased, nostrils flare, throat dilates, air passages dilate – to feed more oxygen to blood.

- The blood thickens, to carry more oxygen and to fight infection, to repair wounds.

- The skin pales, sweats and crawls, hair stands on end, the sense of touch is heightened, as blood is withdrawn, and sweat cools the muscles.

- The senses become acute, pupils dilate, hearing becomes more acute, touch and taste is enhanced.

All this adds up to dramatic change within the body and mind. When we are constantly in a state of readiness, because of our modern lifestyle and the many and varied pressures of family, work and other outside influences, the body adapts, and the switched-on state becomes a new 'normal'. This is called the adaptation response, commonly known as the General Adaptation Response, or GAR.

The perception of a threat is a complex reaction that begins deep in the brain in the amygdala, part of the brain that is on the lookout for danger. In some people this is hyperactive, leading to a constant state of alarm – the sympathetic nervous system doesn't switch off. Add to this the demands of not being able to move quickly, uncertainty as to whether you will be having a good day or a bad day, and the task of following a regime of drugs and any reactions to them, and we can see why stress levels increase with these particular medical conditions.

Identify your stressors

Identifying the factors in life that cause stress can help in planning to overcome it. Recognising the reactions and responses to the situation/person/circumstance is a big step to empowerment and implementing a coping strategy. We can begin simply by making a list of what is stressful, and, within that, what can change and what can't.

Stressors can be divided into different groupings, such as:

- Physical stressors: Environmental factors such as temperature, noise levels, volume of traffic, illness, neighbourhood environment.

- Social, economic and political: Unemployment, financial pressures, housing, level of crime, technological change, health services.

- Family: Domestic workload, jealousy, conflicts caused by social roles, different values, death or illness, different lifestyles, money problems.

- Interpersonal: Differing values, obligations, waiting times, poor service, driving, social expectations.

- Job and career: Deadlines, muddled communications, travelling time, interruptions, power struggles, competition, education/training, bad management.

- Environmental: Pollution, technological change, traffic, overcrowding.

Try making a list of all the stressors you feel affect you negatively. Consider all the categories and see if you need to include something from each of them. Think about your work, health and your private life. Once you have identified the things that make you feel stressed, you are one step nearer to managing them in a more positive way. You can identify whether changes can be implemented, and where things are beyond your power to control, or whether you could do things differently.

Anxiety

People with Parkinson's are susceptible to anxiety – statistics state that over 40 per cent are affected. In yoga terms, this is a Manomaya kosha issue. There are several degrees of anxiety, beginning with GAD, or generalised anxiety disorder. This is an underlying sense that something may go wrong, but this worry has no real basis. Another level, social phobia, is when that persistent worry is related to circumstances in a social context, such as fear of relating to people. A panic attack is when anxiety comes suddenly and with a racing heartbeat, shortness of breath and severe reactions. Anxiety may include low self-esteem, poor coping skills and depression.

Identifying stressors and building a strategy to cope will empower people with Parkinson's or MS. Lowering anxiety levels has the effect of reducing physical symptoms.

What do we mean by relaxation?

The Oxford English Dictionary definition is 'a state of being free from tension and anxiety', which is close to Patanjali's definition of yoga being 'stillness of mind'. Unfortunately, relaxation has become synonymous with anything that is not classed as work, such as listening to music, reading, going for a run even, or watching TV. Today the average life is full, and giving oneself quiet time is a rarity – we are in 'doing' mode most of the time.

In yoga terms, Pratyahara, the fifth of Patanjali's Eight Limbs, equates to relaxing. Meaning 'withdrawal of senses', it suggests that we move our attention away from the stimuli of the external world and focus on the internal experience. Many so-called 'relaxation' practices do not do this, playing music and visualising, while soothing, keeping the mind active and externalised. However, these techniques are useful for some student groups, and provide access to a restful quietness that can be beneficial.

What happens when we relax?

When we begin to relax, the parasympathetic response of the nervous system is engaged, the breath and heart rate slow, and circulation starts to nurture the reproductive system and the digestive system. We relate better to other people, feel warm-hearted and supported. In a relaxed state we can begin to feel more 'normal', able to engage with others, to feel in control and begin to look after ourselves.

Yoga provides a framework for this to happen. By practising the relaxation and breathing techniques on a regular basis, we have a resource when things do not go to plan or we have setbacks. Learning to relax is a vital life-balancing skill. It can be the most healing part of yoga practice, and can begin to undo the negative effects of stress on our physical and mental emotional systems. It needs to be learned and practised, however.

'Relaxation' is used here as a broad term for a variety of techniques. In classical yoga we are used to the term Pratyahara, which is a deep exploration of inner stillness. Practices such as visualisation, affirmation (Pratipaksha Bhavana and Sankalpa, respectively), breath control (Pranayama) and meditation can also bring a relaxed state of being.

This element of yoga practice is an essential aspect in a therapeutic class for students with MS or Parkinson's. Even in an hour-long class, this part of the programme should not be omitted. When choosing a suitable technique, consider the state of awareness of the student, the stage of Parkinson's or MS, and how that may be physically affecting the nervous system.

We experience the world through our nervous system, our senses. We experience our physical body through our nervous system, bearing in mind that the nervous system is greatly affected by both MS and Parkinson's. In MS the electrical message is interrupted, and in Parkinson's the chemical messenger is faulty. This will impact on how a relaxation technique will be perceived by a student.

In my experience it takes a good 20 minutes for the body and the nervous system to settle so that full benefits of relaxation can be felt. A short five minutes listening to a little music will not allow the student to go deep enough into a relaxed state to have any effect on brain wave patterns or parasympathetic system.

In a longer relaxation there is time for a shift in consciousness, and a change in brain wave rhythms from beta to alpha, and for physiological changes to happen. Rigidity in the body and the effect of medication make it difficult to offer the longer relaxation practices such as full yoga nidra. However, much can be achieved with shorter modified versions lasting approximately 15–20 minutes.

How yoga helps

Yoga practice assists in switching on the parasympathetic nervous system to put the break on the stress response and to calm things down. Breathing also plays a big part in this action because of its effect on the vagus nerve, recently identified with emotional stress.

Just managing an illness such as Parkinson's or MS is stressful. Life is governed by drug therapy, and physical limitations impede on activities for both work and play. Joy diminishes. This can start a negative cycle, leading to depression, stress, poor sleep and worsening of physical function, leading to depression, and so on. This also affects people's ability to relate to others and to be able to ask for what they need and to receive help. So relationships deteriorate.

Stress aggravates what would otherwise feel like minor ailments – bad digestion can cause stomach upsets, heartburn and the like, lower immune function means people get more infections, blood pressure gets higher and stays high, impacting on the circulation and blood vessels, increasing the risk of stroke.

WORKING WITH RELAXATION TECHNIQUES

◼ Creating the perfect environment, or doing the best you can

The environment plays a big part in the success of a relaxation practice, and conditions are not always optimal, as rooms/venues, heating systems and general draughtiness vary:

- Temperature: The room should be warm enough for lying still, and/or blankets can be offered. Note that sometimes students with MS prefer a cooler temperature.

- Light: Switch off overhead lighting, but keep some light source on. Don't teach in complete darkness. You must be able to see your students and be able to respond if they become distressed.

- Sound: Although sounds can be soothing, they may trigger emotional responses. Sounds may link into memories and provide stimulus. Musical preferences are very individual – don't assume that what you think is a relaxing piece is heard in the same way by someone else. Silence is golden. Make sure that there are not going to be disturbing noises outside of the room. If there will be noise that cannot be avoided, warn your students.

- Support: The classical Corpse Pose (Savasana) may not be comfortable for everyone. This will depend on rigidity, the shape of the spine and ability to transfer to the floor.

◼ Personal comfort

It is essential that each person is comfortable. This may mean using a different position.

Instruction

1. Start with classical Corpse Pose (Savasana), with a supporting block or two under the head, if needed, paying special attention to the neck position. Kyphosis of the spine will possibly require more blocks or a folded blanket or small pillow. Observe the position of the cervical spine and make sure it is long and not compressed.

2. Legs can be supported with the spine on the mat, knees bent and a chair under the calves and feet, which is helpful if there is a lower back problem, varicose veins or haemorrhoids.

3. The recovery position is useful if there are lower back or other issues that make lying on the spine uncomfortable. Support with a block under the head and possibly under or between knees. Raising the upper body with pillows or bolsters is useful if there are breathing difficulties, depending on which resources you have to hand.

4. If there is no possibility of lying down or getting to the floor, sitting in a chair can work well.

It is helpful to use the same technique until the students are familiar with the practice, leading them gradually into a deeper state. Week by week an 'energetic' path can be created in the psyche. This familiar pattern helps the students to feel safe and to know what is happening. This will facilitate the ability to access deeper levels of relaxation with practice over time. It is important to observe the students while they go through the relaxation practice; you will then pick up if anyone is having difficulties.

Moving into stillness will often bring an emotional response. Take time to comfort anyone who may be feeling emotional. Allow them to sit up, offer a tissue and give them space without fuss, while you continue with the rest of the group session. This will enable them to feel acknowledged without disrupting the class.

Positive vocal input is important. In some ways relaxation is similar to a light hypnotic trance state. Some students (not all) are suggestible, which means that the words used to guide the process are important. Input positive ideas such as:

I breathe in peace.

I am relaxed.

I am warm, comfortable and safe.

Each breath brings balance and harmony that spreads through my whole being.

Moving attention away from external stimulation quietens the mind and students have an opportunity to become quiet and inwardly calm.

■ Squeeze and let go

This is the simplest form and is suitable for those unfamiliar with any relaxation practice. It helps the student to develop focus, concentration and awareness. Tensing and then relaxing muscle groups brings a feeling of control. Experience of the difference between tension and relaxation trains the students in learning how to let go and to know that they can actually do this, and they can take the awareness into their home practice.

Instruction

1. From the feet and working upwards, spread the toes and release.
2. Flex the ankles and point the toes, feeling the stretch in the calves.
3. Tighten the knees – make them feel smaller, then let go.
4. Tighten the thighs, squeeze the buttocks, the pelvic floor – feel them almost lift you off the floor, then let go.
5. Draw in around your waist and suck in your abdomen, as if getting into a tight belt, then let go.
6. Press the shoulder blades into the ground, as if making dents in the floor, then let go.
7. Draw the shoulders across your chest, pull them together, then let go.
8. Lift the arms off the floor, spread the fingers wide, then let go.
9. Make fists, spread the fingers wide, then let go.
10. Lift the head, be aware of tension in the neck, place it back on the floor, then let go.
11. Grit the teeth, then let go.

12. Screw up all of the face, eyes, nose, mouth, then let go.

13. Watch the breathing, how slow and easy it is, rising and falling, rising and falling.

14. Move gently, deepen the breathing and move towards full waking consciousness.

■ Journey through the body

Because of the side effects of medication, it is easy for the Parkinson's students to 'drift off' towards sleep during longer relaxations. Time is needed to take students into a deeper level of relaxation. It is advisable to use the voice to guide the experience and to encourage students to stay awake and focused. A journey through the body will maintain awareness but be enough to lead into a peaceful state while remaining awake and conscious.

As with 'Squeeze and let go', we should follow the same pattern each session, taking the students from a fully conscious state into a quiet calm, 'alpha' state.

Working from the feet to the head gradually draws awareness away from physical experiences to mental quietness and calm, subtle breathing. Even a few minutes in this relaxed state can bring a feeling of calm, refreshed wellbeing. With this inward journey the teacher can encourage the student to explore the shape and form of the physical body through the network of the peripheral nervous system exploring through touch, connecting mind and body.

Outline script

1. Explore the shapes, curves and spaces of your feet, ankles and toes.

2. Move your awareness to the calf and shin; explore and feel the muscle spreading softly. Imagine it filling with golden light, melting any tensions.

3. Explore your knee cap and behind the knee. Imagine golden light pouring around the joint.

4. Let warm light fill the thigh muscle. Explore the top, inside, outside and back of the muscle. Soften the muscle and imagine it sliding away from the bone.

5. Imagine the hip joint having smooth surfaces and pour golden light around it. Imagine the joint loose and free.

6. Move your awareness around to the gluteals and lower back. Feel the muscles spreading layer by layer (add 'Squeeze and let go' if needed).

7. Feel warm golden light spreading through the lower back, as if warmth is coming up from the ground. Let it radiate over the lower back.

8. Explore the connection of your back on the floor, find the hollow places and any areas of tension, breathe into it and let go.

9. Move your awareness up into your shoulder blades and mid-back, back of the neck and across the tops of the shoulders.

10. Move your attention to the front of the body, experience the movement of breath deep in your abdomen, let the waist relax, feel soft in the middle and melt.

11. Feel the rhythm of your breath and the movement of your chest, comfortable, relaxed and easy. Feel warmth around the heart.

12. Be aware of your shoulder joints and imagine softening down into the mat, golden light flowing around the joint. Let go.

13. Be aware of the neck and throat – a swallow can help it relax.

14. Move your attention into the face and the facial muscles; clench the jaw and let go. Let your teeth be apart, let the cheeks fall away, brow clear and smooth, eyelids heavy.

15. Frown and release to help the scalp to relax.

16. Bring awareness into your whole body; with the 'mind's eye' watch the breath.

17. Move deeper into stillness and peace.

It is helpful to keep talking throughout, but use a steady pace and calm voice to assist in holding attention and maintaining concentration.

Coming out of relaxation should be a steady process, not shocking or rushed. The journey inwards was slow and deliberate; the journey out should be considerate of re-engaging with the senses and outside world. I suggest the following order:

1. First of all, bring attention to sounds, listening for sounds nearby, quiet and louder sounds.

2. Then the feel of the breath, the feel of the floor, a sense of touch awakening.

3. Bring attention to the sense of sight, even though the eyes are closed.

4. Then taste and smell.

5. Encourage small movements to reconnect with the physical body and ease into bigger movements and stretching.

6. Encourage the students to tune in to their own bodies to feel how they need to wake up and move.

7. Give warning about any turning on of lights, so that students can be prepared for glare.

8. Give time for everyone to sit up and be fully present and awake.

If anyone is asleep, sitting by them and saying their name will usually wake them; do not shake them.

■ Creating space

A more advanced technique, this takes the student away from the experience of the body. The nervous system is substantially quietened, and efferent nerve messages lessen considerably. The heart rate is lowered and breathing becomes fine and subtle. (This technique may not be useful in the case of the more severely affected students.) In it we create a Zen-like quality of empty space, moving with conscious awareness within the physical body. Use the following order to guide awareness:

Outline script

1. Put your attention in your head and the space within your head. Imagine the area from the right ear to the left ear filling with space.

2. Think of the crown of the head and the tip of the chin; imagine this area filling with space.

3. From the right shoulder to the left shoulder, fill with space.

4. Right shoulder to right hip and left shoulder to left hip, full of space.

5. Right shoulder to left hip and left shoulder to right hip, full of space.

6. Imagine your right arm right down to your wrist, full of space.

7. Fill the left arm with space.

8. Imagine even your fingertips filling with space.

9. From the top of your spine down to the root, fill with space.

10. From your hips to knees and knees to ankles, fill with space.

11. Feel your feet and into your toes filling with space.

12. Be aware of your whole body filled with space.

13. Imagine the space below you, right down through the floor and the earth.

14. Imagine the space above you, up through the ceiling and on out through the atmosphere.

15. Imagine the space to the left.

16. Imagine the space to the right.

17. Feel the space within you and the space outside of you, feel the separation, the boundary of your skin.

18. Imagine the barrier melting away. Be absorbed into a feeling of oneness.

After this practice, take time to bring the students into full awareness, engaging with the solidity of the body, the connection with the earth and sensory function, as described at the end of the 'Journey through the body' technique.

■ Breathing through the body

This technique uses the breath as a focus. Its rhythm induces a state of calm.

Outline script

1. Take your attention to the soles of your feet. Imagine you can breathe through the soles of your feet.

2. As you breathe in, imagine the breath coming up though the soles of your feet like a gentle wave moving up to your ankles and then flowing back down again. Repeat the breath three times.

3. Now breathe in and feel the breath coming up through the soles of your feet and up through your calves to your knees, and then back down as you exhale through the soles of your feet. Repeat three times.

4. On the next inhale, feel the breath flow up to your hips and base of the spine, Muladhara, and then exhale down through your legs and out through your feet. Repeat three times.

5. With your next breath, bring energy up to your waist, Manipura; feel the breath flowing gently up. Let the exhale flow down and out through the soles of your feet. Repeat three times.

6. Feel the flow of energy moving up and down as you breathe.

7. Now bring the breath up past your hips and waist up to the heart, Anahata, in a smooth gentle flow. On the exhales feel the breath flowing down the body and out through the soles of your feet. Repeat three times.

8. On the next inhale bring the breath up past the hips, waist and heart to the throat, Vishuddhi. The out-breath flows down through the whole body and out through the soles of your feet. Repeat three times.

9. The next breath flows all the way up to the brow, Ajna, and down through the throat, heart, waist, hips and legs, out through the feet. Repeat three times.

10. Bring the next inhale all the way up through the whole body to the crown, and breathe out through the whole body through the soles of your feet. Repeat three times.

11. Now we can feel as if the whole body is breathing, the breath being drawn up and down from the feet to the crown and back again.

Let the breath come back to a normal rhythm and bring awareness back into the body and to external awareness.

◼ Resolve (Sankalpa)

Sankalpa is a resolve, a determination that helps us to focus on our goals. It is a positive affirmation, designed to be repeated and to sink into the deep consciousness, until it becomes active and present in waking consciousness. Traditionally, it is meant to strengthen the will, but we have to account for the tricky mental contradiction, intent on sabotaging any hint of reform.

An 'I will' statement puts the action into the future rather than the present; however, in other languages and cultures this may not be the same. 'I am' makes it a present statement it but can be subject to counterproductive critical thought. However, this can be observed and acknowledged and worked through. Alternatively, 'I choose to' could be implemented. Use whichever phrasing feels right for you.

In group terms, a teacher could use a general positive statement, given in the deepest part of the relaxation. Saying to yourself 'I am relaxed', 'I am calm', 'I am safe' would be examples. Otherwise a sankalpa is a deeply personal statement. It may be possible to lead the group in an exploration to find a personal sankalpa, that is meaningful for themselves. Working with a sankalpa or positive affirmation within the relaxation process gives an opportunity to allow the new thought to 'drop' into a deeper state of consciousness. It is thought that as we enter the 'alpha' level of brain wave pattern, we are more receptive to new ideas being implanted, similar to a hypnotic 'suggestion' given in a trance state. These new ideas can then take root, until they grow and manifest in a change of behaviour in the conscious waking state.

◼ Visualisation as a tool for wellbeing

Based on the philosophical idea of 'energy follows thought' or 'as you think, so you become', psychoneuroimmunology is now being taken more seriously and researched. Over the last 50 years or so there have been many books supporting this theory, such as *The Inner Game* (Gallway 1975). This encouraged sports people to spend time on their thought processes as well as improving their physical skills. Psychoneuroimmunology has been researching the effects on the nervous system and the immune system of negative expectations, stress and trauma, showing that positive thoughts boost the immune system. This was famously researched by Candace Pert, American neuroscientist and pharmacologist, who, in 1972, discovered the opiate receptor, the cellular binding site for endorphins in the brain (Pert 1999).

In terms of yoga as a therapy, this concept enhances our practices. Yoga has always been about the union of body and mind. Where we have conflict, we have resistance and struggle, and often set ourselves up to fail. By enhancing the power of the mind, we can progress and build our health in a positive way.

Since the advent of MRI scanning, scientists are able to understand what actually happens in the brain during the thought process, and have discovered that rather than having set pathways, the brain is capable of change, what is now called 'neuroplasticity' – we are capable of building new pathways.

Yoga practices activate energy flow and use the will to establish energy patterns. In yoga nidra, for example, and in other meditative and Pranayama practices, creating energy pathways reinforces the nadis and creates the antakarana (the 'rainbow bridge'), the link between the ego and the higher self/atman or true self.

Visualisation helps to:

- activate positive thinking and influence the function of the hypothalamus and so on to the endocrine system and then body and organ function

- assist concentration in all yoga practices – Asana can be explored more deeply, Pranayama and energy flow are enhanced and mental processes are focused

- establish a positive blueprint for Annamaya kosha, working through Vignanamaya kosha and Pranamaya kosha

- enable us to focus on problem areas, thus gaining an insight into the deeper aspects of the problem and encouraging changes so that the body can heal

- assist with pain relief

- improve mobility

- establish a positive model in many illnesses

- improve creativity

- influence and develop the 'third eye' function at Ajna chakra

- encourage the development of insight and intuition.

The following are some ideas for using the visual process to promote a calming, relaxing mind state. Bear in mind, however, that not everyone has the ability to visualise well. Some people are more oriented to other sensations. Bring in all of the senses, and make sure that people are not expecting to experience full 'technicolour' imagery. These images rely largely on memory as much as imagination.

The following are written as scripts that can be read with pauses to allow time for the imagination.

Go through a short physical awareness relaxation first, to prepare. Some of the images may stir the emotions, so be prepared to offer support.

■ Walking by the sea

Outline script

1. Imagine that you are walking along a seashore; you are in full health and it's a beautiful sunny day. The temperature is just right: warm sunshine, with a gentle breeze.

2. Walk along the beach and feel your feet sinking into the soft, dry sand.

3. Smell the salty sea air, and listen to the sound of the waves coming into shore.

4. There are seabirds overhead and you can hear their calls.

5. Watch the waves coming into the shore, melting into the sand.

6. Walk towards the sea, now walking on the firm, damp sand. Here there is a tide line, where seashells and seaweed are drying in the sun. See the black seaweed drying, the pebbles and shells among the tangle.

7. Stand and look out to sea, your feet sinking a little into the sand.

8. See the sunlight glinting on the water, the white foam on the waves, the colour of the water.

9. Imagine all your worries being taken out to sea on the tide.

10. Enjoy the feel of the sun on your body; breathe in the fresh air.

11. Here the elements are in balance – earth, water, fire and air – promoting a sense of balance within you, recharging your energy and bringing a sense of calm and wellbeing.

12. Turn and walk back up the beach to the warm, soft sand.

13. Let the image melt away, leaving you feeling peaceful and balanced.

■ The light within

The idea of the centre of our being, the home of the true self and the place where Brahman resides within the heart, is found in the Mundaka Upanishad. This philosophical idea can be woven into the relaxation process.

Outline script

1. Move your awareness into your heart space.

2. Imagine moving deeper into the space beyond the realm of the physical heart, deeper than the place of feelings in the emotional heart.

3. Imagine a candle flame here, burning steadily and brightly.

4. Imagine that this place is like a warm, dry cave, with this bright flame at its centre, glowing with a golden light.

5. The flame is bright, giving out its warmth and light.

6. Hold the flame still. It symbolises the eternal part of you. Always there. Radiating light.

7. Be still in this peaceful place.

8. Be.

Come back into full waking consciousness, with full awareness of both yourself and your surroundings.

◼ Walk through the woods in Autumn

Outline script

1. Imagine walking in the woods in Autumn, following a well-worn path, treading the soft earth, damp leaves under your feet.

2. It is a dry sunny day.

3. The trees are clad in their Autumn colours: gold, red, russet and yellow, glowing in the sunlight.

4. Bright berries hang in the trees. Black shiny elderberry clusters. Red rosehips.

5. As you walk, you notice cobwebs hung with water droplets, hanging among the low-lying branches and leaves.

6. Fungi grow out from tree trunks and in clusters on the ground, all different shapes and colours.

7. You notice the damp, earthy woodland smell.

8. Listen to the birdsong and enjoy the rustle of dried leaves as you walk through.

9. Maybe you catch a glimpse of a squirrel darting through the branches.

10. Stand and watch the falling leaves drifting to the earth.

11. Perhaps you are aware of other things on your walk.

12. Turn around and retrace your steps.

13. Enjoy the beauty of nature; let it lift your spirits. Drink in the colour.

14. Feel refreshed and rested.

Come back to full waking consciousness.

■ Therapeutic visualising

We can devise personal positive imaging for individual needs. For example, the person who has spasticity or rigidity in the feet could be encouraged to visualise that these unwilling parts of the body are moving freely, and there is fluidity of movement and space between the joints, so that they can visualise their feet flexing and pointing, opening and closing. This can be done along with attempted movement or without.

We can bring this idea into any area that is tight and immobile, visualising how it would be if it was elastic and soft and what a difference that would make to mobility and life in general. If working one-to-one, we can tailor the imaging to the needs of the student, agreeing on images and language that work for them.

In group Yoga Therapy we can offer more general exercises that are individualised by the student's experience. The results may be discussed in the group, and shared to deal with the difference between the visualisation and reality, if time allows.

■ Body strength and stability

This can be a powerful exercise and may bring up an emotional response. Be ready to witness the feelings and acknowledge them rather than stopping the process. It's okay to cry, to feel.

Outline script

1. Imagine you are going on a country walk. You begin by climbing a hill, following a defined path.

2. The climb is easy and your body feels strong. Enjoy that feeling.

3. You stride out at a good pace, planting your feet firmly on the ground. There is ease and grace in your walk; it feels good.

4. You make good progress and are breathing comfortably.

5. Your shoulders are relaxed and your arms swing in time with your stride.

6. You reach the crest of the hill. You feel strong and full of energy. Feel the earth solid under your feet, and imagine drawing that strength up into your body.

7. What does that feel like?

8. From this viewpoint you can see the land spreading out, like a patchwork quilt.

9. Breathe deeply.

10. Turn to walk back down the hill.

11. You walk with ease and confidence. Your feet feel safe on the path.

■ Control room

This is a process that is left 'open' in some parts to let the students explore themselves.

Outline script

1. Connect into the centre of your being, the place where your higher self dwells – you might feel that this is in your head or in your heart.

2. Imagine that you are in a control room. All around you are dials and levers that control your life.

3. You find a dial that is a stress indicator. Look at the reading and turn it down.

4. You find a dial that is for strength; you can turn that up a little.

5. There may be other dials showing 'fear' or 'patience'.

6. What else can you see? Make the adjustments that will help you.

7. Explore the control room and adjust any dials that are showing readings that you would like to change.

8. You can return at any time to adjust the settings.

■ Clearing the pranic body (Aluloma Vilima Kriya)

Alu refers to the pranic body. This is a practice to balance energy flow and the pranas of the vital body. It can be used as a deep relaxation technique. It provides psychic protection and helps to ward off negative thoughts and the disturbing energies of other people.

Instruction

1. Lie in Corpse Pose (Savasana) (see page 229).

2. Steady your breathing and practise Savitri Pranayama to a 8:4:8:4 rhythm for five rounds.

3. Imagine lying in a large oval of energy, which extends above your head and below your feet. It is two halves, one to the right and one to the left.

4. Visualise energy flowing down the left curve of the oval, from above your head to below your feet, on the exhale breath. Hold for a moment. Then feel energy rising up the right side, from below your feet to above your head, on the inhale breath.

5. Complete nine rounds of ovaling the energy.

6. Now imagine the oval starting at the crown and reaching to the feet. Oval the energy as before, using the breath. Complete nine rounds.

7. Now restrict the oval to a point within the centre of the brain (Ajna) and the base of the spine (Muladhara). Breathing out down the left curve, Apana flowing down, Ajna to Muladhara. Breathing in, up the right curve from Muladhara to Ajna, prana flowing up. Complete nine rounds.

8. The practice can continue to focus on energy moving in the narrow loop of Ida (left) and Pingala (right) nadis.

9. After the practice, gently shift awareness to the senses and outside world.

10. Move slowly, ground and stretch.

Managing pain the yoga way

Orthodox view of pain and its treatment

In 'Insights into pain: A review of qualitative research', Mike Osborn and Karen Rodham (2010) say:

> The very nature of pain (subjective, dynamic and multi-dimensional) means it is extremely difficult to quantify… Qualitative approaches attempt to explore the personal experience of [pain]… A range of studies focused on the lived experience of a number of pain conditions… [C]hronic pain was the most commonly researched type of pain…
>
> Of prime importance was the feeling expressed by patients that others did not recognise the practical and emotional issues that participants experienced as they dealt with their pain condition in the context of their 'normal everyday' lives. In particular, the participants' accounts showed that they often shared: feelings of confusion and worry; an ongoing assault on the self by the pain, and the social and cultural unpleasantness of living with pain.

This study noted that despite usually living with their pain for many years, the participants were often confused about their pain and, as they couldn't make sense of it, were worried about their future. The following quotes show the nature of the despair related to pain:

> 'It is there all the time…it's just, I just want to know what…what the pain is.'
>
> '…you know, coping with pain is one thing, but coping with the psychological thing is really hard.'
>
> '…surely it can only get worse…'

Kathy Charmaz, in 'Loss of self: A fundamental form of suffering in the chronically ill' (1983), described a similar process where pain produced a 'fundamental loss of self'. Pain appeared to stifle communication: '…some people must think I whinge and I try and when they say "how are you?" I say "fine".'

Charmez goes on to say:

> This paper has provided a summary of qualitative empirical work that has been published over the last ten years. This research has focused both on the experience and process of managing pain. We demonstrated that people who live with pain also live with confusion and worry as they try to make sense of what they feel is an uncertain future. People living with pain spoke of the struggle to maintain a sense of identity whilst dealing with the additional problems of maintaining normal social and familial roles. The experience of living with pain was coloured by the process of seeking help to manage their pain. There was a strong sense of hopelessness and distress from both those living with pain, and the health professionals providing support. Thus, as we

noted above, qualitative research demonstrates that pain is something which extends beyond the sensory and cognitive domains, to foreground the destructiveness of the interpersonal, social and cultural factors involved.

These observations may also apply to those with an ongoing long-term illness.

Pain gate theory

Defining terms:

- Pain is an unpleasant sensory and emotional experience associated with actual or potential tissue damage.

- Analgesia is the selective suppression of pain without effects on consciousness or other sensations.

- Nociceptors are sensory receptors whose stimulation causes pain.

- Pain threshold is the point at which a stimulus is perceived as painful.

- Sensation is the process of receiving, converting and transmitting information from the external and internal world to the brain.

Melzack and Wall described gate control theory in 1965. This theory explains about a pain-modulating system in which a neural gate present in the spinal cord can open and close, thereby modulating the perception of pain. The gate control theory suggests that psychological factors play a role in the perception of pain.

The three systems located in the spinal cord acting to influence the perception of pain are:

- the substantia gelatinosa in the dorsal horn

- the dorsal column fibres

- the central transmission cells.

The noxious impulses are influenced by a 'gating mechanism'. Stimulation of the large-diameter fibres inhibits the transmission of pain, thus 'closing the gate', whereas when smaller fibres are stimulated, the gate is opened. When the gate is closed, signals from small-diameter pain fibres do not excite the dorsal horn transmission neurons. When the gate is open, pain signals excite dorsal horn transmission cells. The gating mechanism is influenced by nerve impulses that descend from the brain.

Factors that influence *opening* and *closing* the gate are:

- the amount of activity in the pain fibres

- the amount of activity in other peripheral fibres

- messages that descend from the brain.

The gate is opened by:

- physical factors – bodily injury

- emotional factors – anxiety and depression

- behavioural factors – attending to the injury and concentrating on the pain.

The gate may be closed by:

- physical pain – analgesic remedies

- emotional pain – being in a 'good' mood

- behavioural factors – concentrating on things other than the injury.

This theory helps to explain how interventions based on somatosensory (auditory, visual and tactile) stimulation such as friction, music therapy and distraction provide pain relief. On this basis we can see how yoga practice would help relieve pain.

In the UK the NHS website suggests self-help under the following headings:

'Get some gentle exercise'

'Breathe right'

'Stay positive'

'Distract yourself'

'Get some sleep'

'Socialise'

'Relax.' (NHS Choices, n.d.)

Pain is usually described as 'acute', a largely short-lived and temporary experience, or 'chronic', long-term and ongoing. Pain is processed in the brain. Chronic pain causes the brain to change, and it is now thought that we can change this experience, as the brain has neuroplastic properties. A definition of neuroplasticity is: 'The capacity of neurons and neural networks in the brain to change their connections and behaviour in response to new information, sensory stimulation, development, damage or dysfunction' (Encyclopaedia Britannica).

We can begin this process using:

- Asana

- mindful movement

- autonomic nervous system regulation

- meditation

- Bhavana

- memory.

Key areas of the brain involved in experiencing pain are as follows:

- Amygdala: Processes emotions, fear, anger, pleasure, memory.

- Hippocampus: Memory, spatial navigation, short-term to long-term memory. Patients with depression, post-traumatic stress disorder and chronic pain all have atrophy of the hippocampus (impaired memory; see Rubenstein and Roseman 2011).

- Thalamus: Processes sensory input and directs it to appropriate areas of the brain. Atrophies in chronic pain. Meditation shows a difference in thalamic activity (Kigi 2005).

- Somatosensory cortex: Areas of the body are mapped in the brain. Pain causes the sensory cortex to expand and motor cortex to reduce; movement stimulates blood flow in the brain or reduces it.

- Prefrontal cortex: The area dealing with emotion and learning. In chronic pain, the memory of pain gets 'stuck', causing prolonged activity in this area.

Managing pain the yoga way

Many with Parkinson's and MS are familiar with pain to varying degrees. It is worthwhile building into any therapeutic yoga programme techniques that may lessen the experience of pain.

In relation to the five koshas, sensory intensity, location and quality of pain is an Annamaya experience. Emotional responses are Manomaya. Cognitive thoughts related to pain experience are both Manomaya and Vijnanamaya.

It is also worth bearing in mind that the intensity of the pain is not indicative of the severity of the problem; for example, a paper cut is very painful, but we may not notice the presence of a tumour.

Patanjali tells us in Sutra 2.33, 'When disturbed by negative thoughts, opposite thoughts should be thought of.' This is known as Pratipaksha Bhavana. We are also guided in the following Sutras:

- Sutra 1.34 – calm is retained by the controlled exhalation or retention of the breath.

- Sutra 1.35 – concentration on subtle sense perception can cause steadiness of the mind.

METHODS FOR REDUCING PAIN

▓ Method 1: Body scan

Taking time to move your awareness around the body in a methodical way can help to reduce the sensations of pain. Rather than feeling overwhelmed by pain, we are able to acknowledge that this painful feeling resides in a particular place and that we can choose to move awareness to a different place.

Instruction

1. Be comfortable and slow down your breathing.

2. Focus your attention in your feet and notice any sensations there – everything is welcome; try not to label things as good or bad.

3. Gradually move your awareness through your body, part by part. Let go of anything other than what you are experiencing. Stay completely in the present moment.

4. Move into a place of awareness of the whole body, of breath and stillness.

▓ Method 2: Positive thinking (Pratipaksha Bhavana)

In her book *Yoga for Pain Relief*, Kelly McGonigal (2009) suggests the following practice:

1. Start with where you are, allow yourself to feel the feelings. What is happening in your mind and body right now? Notice sensations, thoughts and emotions.

2. Take a little time to accept what you are feeling. When you are no longer resisting, move to the next step.

3. Ask yourself: If I were completely free of this pain (stress fatigue, anger, fear, etc.) what would I be thinking or feeling instead? What state of mind and body would heal what I am feeling right now? The answer will become the focus of your meditation – comfort, warmth, energy, acceptance, forgiveness, gratitude, courage, etc.

4. Bring in a memory or image of how that state feels. You can use, colours, sounds, a person or anything that inspires the feeling. Let the body sensations that go with this state wash over your mind and body.

5. Stay with the process as long as you like.

6. Come back to the present moment, and let go of any attempt to control what you are thinking or feeling. Acknowledge to yourself that you have the strength to handle all sensations and you are free to choose healing and balance.

■ Method 3: Visualisation 1

This uses the creative power of the mind to minimise the experience of pain.

Instruction

1. Visualise the area of the body that hurts, and describe what you see.

2. How might you change this? What would you like to happen?

3. Visualise step-by-step changes until there is complete change (visualised).

4. How have the pain levels changed?

■ Method 4: Visualisation 2

Giving the pain size and a quantity helps us to explore its limits and empowers us to change it, using creative thinking.

Instruction

1. The teacher proposes that the pain has mass – how big is it? What would it fit into? Start with a suggested container – it could be anything from a pint jug to a skip! Define this (it is a way of you being able to express how your pain feels to you).

2. Imagine pouring the pain into a smaller container, just the next size down. Pour the pain.

3. Go smaller and smaller until there is only a thimbleful. This can be poured away.

4. Think about the pain levels you experience and compare them.

5. Work with Vijnanamaya. Pain is a warning signal; its purpose is to alert the body that all is not well. To understand its impact, it may help to have an imagined dialogue with the pain to understand its purpose. This could be playful, an experiment. It doesn't have to be done 'correctly'.

6. It might be led in the following way:

   What does your pain look like? 'A small red dragon.'

   Does the dragon have anything to say? 'Take notice of me.'

   I am certainly aware of you, do you have a purpose? 'To make you stop/slow down.'

   How can I do that? (A possible solution or helpful insight may occur here.)

   Thank you, dragon.

This may seem trivial but it can help to identify changes to be made.

Chakra practices

When using the chakras in Yoga Therapy work, there are several considerations:

1. Is the student familiar and comfortable working in this way? If they have never done yoga before, the whole idea may seem very foreign and incomprehensible to them, like a foreign language that you would have to teach from the beginning.

2. What is your goal for working this way?

3. What are your expectations and outcomes for the client/student?

The chakra system is a subtle energy system with its roots in Tantra Yoga. It has a symbolic language showing its connections to the flow of prana and relating to mental and emotional states, both positive and negative. The position of centres along the spine relates to the nerve plexuses and there is also a connection to the endocrine system, creating a physical connection. These energy centres are thought to have a level of function in the physical body as an underlying 'life energy'. When this flow of prana is disturbed, ill health will eventually follow. Prana is disturbed by thoughts and feelings, especially if they become habitual, as in trauma or continuing negative thought patterns.

If disease manifests in the physical body, it is usually at the stage where it needs physical intervention and treatment, be that a physical practice, surgery or medication. Working on the chakras alone will have little or no impact on the physical level.

It is at the emotional level that we can successfully promote change. If we identify and remove or lessen the mental/emotional disturbance, we can allow energy to flow more freely.

We can use chakra symbolism, as colour, shape and sound, to connect with the subtle energy level in the centre on which we are focusing.

The world of research has yet to take the subject seriously enough to warrant a proper study, but a minor study from G. Hogan, studying with the Australian Institute of Yoga Therapy and the Centre for Adult Education, and under the supervision of Dr Angela Hass, Melbourne, Australia (2009), indicated that chakra focus provided a revitalisation of the individual's health, physically, mentally and emotionally.

Asana can begin to work the physical areas of the spine related to each chakra and bring awareness to the physical area of influence, but the major part of chakra work will be through breathing and meditation.

First, we have to bring a knowledge of this system to the fore. It is a detailed and complex body of knowledge, but we can begin by simply explaining the seven centres as a focus, using breathing as the conduit. You do not need to use the Sanskrit words – the location terminology will be more understandable for the average class member or therapy student.

Those who have worked with me know that I am a traditionalist; where colour and chakras are concerned, I link these with the elements and the pranas, not the rainbow.

■ Chakra awareness exercise 1

Instruction

1. Begin by focusing on the movement of breath in your heart. This is your heart chakra; watch the breath here for a few moments.

2. Imagine you are going to draw a line from your heart to your throat; it will rise like a line of light, like the fluid in a thermometer. See it flowing up and down, from the heart centre up to the throat centre as you breathe in, and from the throat to the heart as you breathe out. Do this for five breaths.

3. On the next exhale, extend the line down to your navel, and then continue breathing up from your navel through the heart and up to the throat, connecting navel, heart and throat centres. Keep breathing along the line.

4. Now extend the line down into the centre of the sacrum on the next exhale, and again draw it up from the sacral centre up through the navel, and from the heart to the throat. Let the breath rise and fall, connecting the centres.

5. As you inhale, bring the next breath up to the brow, then breathe out all the way down to the sacral. Keep breathing along this extended line through the navel, heart and throat, to the brow.

6. Finally, breathe all the way up to the crown of your head on the in-breath and all the way down to the base of the spine on the out-breath. The breath connects all of the energy centres.

7. Come back to the heart and watch your breath in your heart for a little time.

8. Move your awareness outwards and become aware of your surroundings.

■ Chakra awareness exercise 2

This can be done lying in Corpse Pose (Savasana) (see page 229) or sitting.

Instruction

1. Root, Muladhara: The site of Muladhara can easily be experienced through the action of contracting and releasing the perineum. We can think of the root or base centre as being here. Visualise that you are breathing in a warm feeling of strength into this place as if you are drawing it coming up through the ground. This will help the connection into the earth and its qualities of strength and patience. Imagine it growing in intensity, at the bottom of the spine. Do this for five breaths. The symbol of a yellow square could be visualised here. The square represents the earth, solid, firm and steady, supporting everything; bring those qualities into the root.

2. Sacral, Swadhistana: Move your awareness up from the root chakra into the centre of the pelvis, the sacral centre. Feel as if you are bringing in a sense of warmth that flows up into this area. This is a liquid warmth, fluid and sensuous. Feel the warmth filling the pelvis. Do this for five breaths. The symbol of a white crescent moon could be visualised here, a symbol of water, nourishing and bringing life, fluid and yet powerful. Bring those qualities into the sacral space.

3. Navel, Manipura: Move your awareness to the level of your navel. Imagine breathing into this place, drawing in a warmth that circulates around your stomach and solar plexus. Imagine a glowing ball of energy in your middle like a sun. A red inverted triangle could be visualised here; it is the symbol of fire, bringing light, warmth and energy; feel those qualities coming into the your navel centre.

4. Heart, Anahata: Move your awareness to the level of your heart. Feel your breath moving easily into this centre as if you are drawing it horizontally into your heart. Feel a warm, comforting glow in the heart, and let it spread around your chest. A smokey blue hexagon could be visualised here. The hexagon represents the element of air, invisible and multidirectional; it brings sensitivity. We experience it through touch; it connects us to our feelings and sustains life through breath.

5. Throat, Visuddhi: Move your awareness up to your throat. Imagine breathing energy down into your throat, a cooler feeling, clear and fine. Let it spread around your throat and voice. A white circle could be visualised here. This is the symbol for space or ether, and connects with sound and hearing. Through communication we begin to understand, connect and express ourselves. Feel that breathing here will help the power of communication.

6. Brow, Ajna: Move your awareness into the centre of your forehead just between your eyebrows where you would imagine your mind's eye to be. Keep your attention focused here for five breaths. A two-petalled lotus could be visualised here. Here we connect with the function of the mind and intellect, the quality of wisdom and understanding. Allow the breath to bring a balanced calm as symbolised by the two petals.

7. Crown, Sahasrara: Bring your attention to the crown of your head and keep your attention focused here; be aware of any sensations that you notice, for five breaths. Feel that you are moving to a place of light, a sense of spirituality can be contacted here.

8. Guide your consciousness all the way back down to the base of your spine, and then out into your body.

9. Feel the movement of your breath and begin to wriggle your fingers and toes. Stretch and move, and sit up in your own time.

CHAKRA WORK WITH THE INDIVIDUAL

■ Chakra diagnostics

To diagnose the function of the chakra energy in any individual means spending time not only finding out what physical symptoms are present, but also, more usefully, finding out more about the emotional states. In Chapter 2 there is an overview of how diseases like Parkinson's and MS will impact on the mental and emotional state, but each person has a different emotional make-up. This will be a rich mix of their beliefs, experiences, cultural and social influences, as well as their current situation. It will take time to build up a picture of the function and pattern of the subtle energy.

■ Annamaya level, physical

The location and origins of the physical symptoms of illness in the body will indicate the chakra that is most out of balance. For undiagnosed symptoms, observe where the discomfort is experienced and locate the nearest chakra.

- Muladhara: Issues with walking and standing, problems affecting the legs, feet and bones. Health issues concerning the function of elimination, such as haemorrhoids and constipation. Ailments of the lower pelvis and bowel. Adrenals. Problems with the sense of smell.

- Swadhistana: Problems of the reproductive system, gonads, kidneys and urinary tract, and balance of fluids in the body. Problems with the sense of taste.

- Manipura: Digestive problems, stomach, liver, gall bladder and pancreas, and illnesses that concern the functioning of these organs, such as diabetes. General low-energy states.

- Anahata: Heart and lungs, respiratory and circulatory problems, thymus, immune system. Shoulders, arms and hands. Asthma, breathing difficulties, blood pressure issues.

- Visuddhi: Problems with swallowing or speaking. Thyroid problems, neck and throat. Problems with hearing.

- Ajna: Cognitive difficulties, function of the brain. Pineal and pituitary. Faulty thought processes. Brain chemistry imbalances.

- Sahasrara: Physical symptoms would not manifest here.

■ Pranamaya level, energy flow (see Prana vayus in Chapter 2)

Ask about overall energy levels and quality of sleep. Check breathing function.

- Muladhara: Apana, downward-flowing energy and downward-flowing functions.

- Swadhistana: Apana, down-flowing function such as menstruation and giving birth, and samana, in that the digestive organs fill this area and the absorption of energy continues through the intestinal tract.

- Manipura: Samana, supports digestion and creation of energy, vyana supports overall nourishment.

- Anahata: Vyana, circulatory function and prana movement of breath and life-bringing energy.

- Visuddhi: Udana, upward-flowing, supporting the senses and brain processes.

- Ajna: Udana.

- Sahasrara: All.

■ Manomaya level, lower mind

Ask questions to discern the emotional state of the student, and find how these relate to the chakras.

Identify positive qualities that will enable you to build a picture of both their strengths and frailties.

The following is a brief outline of negative emotional patterns that would disturb the flow of energy, suggestions for questions that may reveal issues, and positive qualities for each chakra.

Muladhara

- Negatives are feeling unsafe; over-concern with the material world and accumulating possessions, which stems from fear of loss; feeling that the world is a threatening place; not being able to stand up for yourself.

- Positives are strong and steadfast, patient, organised and secure.

- Do you feel safe and secure? Do you feel supported and provided for? Can you trust the future? Do you feel you belong?

Swadhistana

- Negatives are over-emotional; lacking creative outlets; feelings of inadequacy; feeling powerless and unfulfilled; jealous; indulgent behaviour; easily manipulated by others or being manipulative; erratic temperament.

- Positives are creative; able to go with the flow; adaptable.

- Do you feel financially secure? Are you flexible or too easily manipulated? Are there any issues concerning sexuality?

Manipura

- Negatives are lack of self-worth; anger at being neglected; lack of confidence; pent-up emotion.

- Positives are self-confident; enthusiastic; able to digest ideas and facts as well as food.

- Do you feel valued? Are you frightened of getting it wrong? Do you worry what others will think?

Anahata

- Negatives are feeling unloved and unlovable; feeling overwhelmed by emotion; emotional hurt and pain; grief; lack of joy; selfishness.

- Positives are compassionate; loving; fair.

- Are you able to express love for others or does fear of rejection hold you back? Do you feel loved and lovable?

Visuddhi

- Negatives are unable to speak out and express your own views; feeling unheard; not able to express emotions, choking back feelings; unable to express creativity.

- Positives are feeling in control; able to express oneself with clarity; creative.

- Are you able to speak the truth? Do you express your creativity?

Ajna

- Negatives are confusion, not able to think or see clearly; feeling fuzzy-headed; muddled perception; tendency to intellectualise things; feeling uninspired.

- Positives are clear thinking; perceptive; open to new ideas; intuitive.

- Do you get confused and muddled? Do you follow your hunches? Do you overthink things?

Sahasrara

- Negatives are not feeling connected spiritually; feeling conflicted about religious beliefs.

- Positives are feeling spiritually connected and inspired, at one; joy in being.

- There are questions about beliefs and any conflicts arising, for example, feeling angry with God often arises in cases of chronic illness.

◼ Vignanamaya level, wisdom

Only when we are able to recognise our stuck places and see them differently do we enter the realm of wisdom. Then we are able to plan new strategies, see life from a different perspective and move forward. This enables us to free ourselves from kleshas and samskaras. This will happen only slowly, but when it does, there is an acceptance and contentment, whatever our physical state of being.

◼ Anandamaya level, bliss

This level links to feelings of joy, love, inspiration and spirituality. Encouraging students to look for beauty in nature, or to find pleasure in the mundane, may help to boost the chakra energy at this finest of the koshas – for example, love of the outdoors walks will boost the Muladhara energy.

When working with the chakras, we are looking to find a balance within the whole system. Working with only one centre will create imbalance, just as in asana practice we would not think of only practising one posture. If you are working therapeutically to clear and balance one particular centre, work to balance the whole system to complete the work.

In general, working with Parkinson's and MS students, the common problems will be in the lower chakras, so establishing awareness throughout these centres will bring life, strength and balance for these students.

CHAKRA PRACTICES IN GENERAL

▓ Muladhara practices

Asana: Standing postures, Warrior Poses, standing balances, Cobbler Pose, and one-leg fold (Janu Sirshasana). Allow 10–15 minutes for visualisation.

Instruction

1. Imagine standing on the earth, like a tree growing, roots deep down. Feel as if you are bringing energy up from the ground into your base chakra.

2. Use your breath and imagine drawing up strength and energy, up through the roots.

3. What colour is this energy? Let it fill your legs and spread through your toes, flowing up, into your lower abdomen and lower back.

4. Let go of fear on the exhale breath; imagine it being absorbed by the earth.

5. Feel strong and courageous.

Images such as caves, digging in gardens, finding buried treasure, sensations of walking on gravel or soft sand, and earthy scents – these can all help to connect with the Muladhara chakra.

Affirmations:

> I have all the strength I need.
>
> I am safe and provided for.
>
> I trust life.

Take time to let your student work out the wording that they feel fits their need.

▓ Swadhistana practices

Asana: Seated Forward Bend (Paschimottanasana), Cobra Pose, Locust Pose, hip stretches. Allow 10–15 minutes for visualisation.

Instruction

1. Imagine the lower half of your body filled with water, like a clear, calm lake.

2. Imagine sitting by the water, watching it lapping; sometimes a strong wind will whip up the surface and it becomes choppy.

3. Wait until it becomes calm again.

4. Imagine a pale bright moon rising in the sky and you see this reflected perfectly on the surface of the water. Know that when the waters become stormy you can calm them.

5. Be aware of the life-giving qualities of water. It nourishes the land and promotes growth and life.

6. This centre is where life begins. Breathe in nourishment, fluidity, adaptability, and breathe out jealousy and feelings of 'stuckness'.

Images such as floating or being by the sea, rivers and pools, tasting things such as juicy fruits – these will connect with this chakra.

Affirmations:

> I am nurtured and supported.
>
> I go with the flow.
>
> I am abundant and prosperous.
>
> I turn my ideas into reality.
>
> I allow pleasure and sweetness in my life.

■ Manipura practices

Asana: All twisting postures, Standing Forward Bend (Uttanasana), Cat Pose. Allow 10–15 minutes for visualisation.

Instruction

1. Imagine sitting by a campfire. The ground is firm, but you are comfortable. You can feel the warmth of the fire on your skin. The warmth permeates your whole body.

2. Look into the flames, see the flickering shapes and colours, and the glowing embers; the flames burn brightly, yellow and gold; sometimes you see greens and blues in the flames.

3. Occasionally, sparks fly up with wisps of smoke into the air. The fire creates both warmth and light.

4. Watch the flickering light and shadows it creates.

Images of candle flames, fire, the sun and receiving sunlight help us to connect with Manipura. Breathe in courage, self-confidence, and breathe out fatigue, fears and anger.

Affirmations:

> I have all the energy I need.
>
> I am secure in who I am.

■ Anahata practices

Asana: Back-bending postures, welcome breath, shoulder-opening stretches. Allow 10–15 minutes for visualisation.

Instruction

1. Bring your attention into your heart and imagine a pink rose in bud.

2. Keep your attention here, and allow the bud to begin to open – one by one, the petals part.

3. Look at the colour of the flower and the soft petals. See it open more with each breath that you take.

4. You might think of all the people that you love and allow the rose to open with that feeling. Imagine a drop of dew caught between the petals, sparkling like a diamond.

5. As the rose opens, you can smell the lovely delicate perfume, carried on the air. This is a symbol of the unseen spiritual presence in the heart.

6. Move closer to the flower and feel the touch of the petals on your skin, soft and delicate. Let the flower close slowly.

Use images focused in the heart and engaging, warm, loving feelings, being open-hearted, generous compassionate and kind – images involving the sense of touch, the feel of velvet, stroking a pet, for example.

Affirmations:

I both give and receive love.

I find joy in my life.

I am compassionate for myself and others.

■ Vishuddhi practices

Asana: Neck rotations, Bridge Pose, mantra, 'legs up the wall'. Allow 10–15 minutes for visualisation.

Instruction

1. Feel the flow of air in your throat.

2. Imagine a circle of white and that you are bringing clarity and light into the throat space.

3. Listen to inner sounds.

Use images of open space, evening sky with stars, being in high places with the sound of the wind.

Affirmations:

I speak my truth.

I communicate clearly.

I am heard.

I express my creativity.

◼ Ajna practices

Asana: Alternate nostril breathing, meditation, Child Pose. Visualisation: do seven rounds of 'breathing'. Visualisation itself stimulates Ajna and engages the will and power of the mind.

Instruction

1. Visualise alternate nostril breathing without using your hands, but by mentally directing the breath up through the left nostril to the space between the brows, and then flowing it down through the right nostril.

2. Reverse the process.

3. Imagine that you are drawing an inverted 'V' as you do this.

Affirmations:

My mind is clear.

My thoughts are calm.

I trust my intuition.

◼ Sahasarara practices

Making a spiritual connection is a supportive act, enhancing quality of life, joy and contentment and the ability to step out of the everyday to look at the wider aspects of humanity. It is often reported that people with a strong faith find that they are happier. It is this aspect of the crown centre that could be considered therapeutic. It may not be in the scope of a therapeutic class to explore this aspect of life, but there may be opportunity to present it as a topic for discussion. Allow 10–15 minutes for visualisation.

Instruction

1. We can begin to create awareness of this centre by bringing our breath up to the crown in the area of the fontanelle, and observing any sensations that occur.

2. Imagine the breath coming up and out through the crown of the head, like a fountain.

3. The fountain of sparkling light flows down and around the body, cascading over the shoulders, down the spine, and over the front of your body, as if you are sitting in the midst of a fountain of light. The light shimmers with all the colours of the rainbow.

4. Let the image fade away and feel that the crown centre is closing like the lens of a camera.

Always complete any chakra work by balancing the whole system, using Chakra Shuddhi with the intention of balancing throughout the whole system.

■ Short Chakra Shuddhi practice (purification)

Instruction

1. Take your attention down to Muladhara at the base of the spine, and focus your breath in this centre. Direct your breath as if you are breathing in and out of the centre, with the intention to clear and balance. Affirm: 'I am clearing and balancing Muladhara chakra.' Repeat seven times.

2. Take your attention down to Swadhistana at the sacrum, and focus your breath in this centre. Direct your breath as if you are breathing in and out of the centre, with the intention to clear and balance. Affirm: 'I am clearing and balancing Swadhistana chakra.' Repeat seven times.

3. Take your attention to Manipura at the navel, and focus your breath in this centre. Direct your breath as if you are breathing in and out of the centre, with the intention to clear and balance. Affirm: 'I am clearing and balancing Manipura chakra.' Repeat seven times.

4. Take your attention into Anahata in the heart, and focus your breath in this centre. Direct your breath as if you are breathing in and out of the centre, with the intention to clear and balance. Affirm: 'I am clearing and balancing Anahata chakra.' Repeat seven times.

5. Take your attention to Vishuddhi at the throat, and focus your breath in this centre. Direct your breath as if you are breathing in and out of the centre, with the intention to clear and balance. Affirm: 'I am clearing and balancing Vishuddhi chakra.' Repeat seven times.

6. Take your attention to Ajna in the brow, and focus your breath in this centre. Direct your breath as if you are breathing in and out of the centre, with the intention to clear and balance. Affirm: 'I am clearing and balancing Ajna chakra.' Repeat seven times.

7. Take your attention up to Sahasarara at the crown, and focus your breath in this centre. Direct your breath as if you are breathing in and out of the centre, with the intention to clear and balance. Affirm: 'I am clearing and balancing Sahasrara chakra.' Repeat seven times.

8. Bring awareness back down the spine, stopping briefly with a thought of balance for each chakra, so that on completing the practice, awareness is in the root rather than the crown. This will encourage groundedness rather than a light-headed 'out of it' state.

9. Breathing can be shortened to three or five repeats to fit the time you have. It is better to do a shortened version rather than none at all, so that the student feels balanced and complete.

Meditation

It is currently popular to use the word 'mindfulness' when referring to meditation practices, and much research has been made into the positive health effects using the 'rediscovered' mindfulness techniques, although, in essence, it is a practice that has been known for a long time. It is present in the yoga tradition and the effects on health and wellbeing are the same. Researchers have been very active in showing the benefits of meditation and mindfulness for improved mental health, and for help in dealing with depression and stress.

In 2014, Madhav Goyal, an assistant professor in the Division of General Internal Medicine at the Johns Hopkins University School of Medicine, along with colleagues, published 'Meditation programs for psychological stress' (Goyal *et al.* 2014). The research found that 'Some 30 minutes of meditation daily may improve symptoms of anxiety and depression'. 'A lot of people use meditation, but it's not a practice considered part of mainstream medical therapy for anything,' says Goyal. 'But in our study, meditation appeared to provide as much relief from some anxiety and depression symptoms as what other studies have found from antidepressants... These patients did not typically have full-blown anxiety or depression.' The researchers evaluated the degree to which those symptoms changed in people who had a variety of medical conditions, such as insomnia or fibromyalgia, although only a minority had been diagnosed with a mental illness.

In everyday life our mind becomes full; we are more often than not disturbing ourselves with troubled thoughts and worries, 'to do' lists and responsibilities. Add to the mix illness and medication, clinic appointments and generally managing one's life, and we can soon become overloaded. Many people with Parkinson's and MS are working and managing their health alongside family and business. This can tip them over the edge into full-on clinical depression and anxiety.

Meditation is one of the most therapeutic practices that we can offer, although it does take application. A contradictory note is that ill health is one of the obstacles to practice, as stated in Patanjali's Sutras. That being so, quietening the mind has a calming effect on the nervous system and can help to bring things into a new perspective. Making these shifts can bring a strength and ability to cope. We may start to realise that we are not the mind, nor the emotions, but that these things will pass and that we have a choice on how we respond and react to many everyday situations.

Meditation offers an oasis of calm in a busy life and can help to alleviate physical symptoms that are often made worse by stress. Meditation practice can be taught in small bites. The first step is to develop concentration, the sixth of the 'Eight Limbs', Dharana.

Before embarking on teaching meditation to others it is essential to experience it for yourself. I know that some yoga trainings do not focus on meditation, so it would be wise to practise and become familiar with what happens, and with the kind of progress that you can expect and obstacles that you may meet.

When thinking of using meditation as a therapeutic tool, we must first consider whether it is suitable for the student/client. If your student/client is a yoga practitioner, it will not be a problem, but with a student who is unfamiliar with yoga's wide scope, the practices have to be introduced step by step.

It is helpful to:

- Explain the process in lay terms.

- Train focus and concentration, just as you would in a beginner's yoga class, using objects, breath, etc. and working from the tangible focus with an object, to the intangible abstract ideas.

- Move on to the subject matter that is therapy-focused. This might be chakra-based breath, using words, sounds or images.

The meditation practice should have a clear method, with attention to:

- sitting comfortably and preparation

- breathing

- a therapeutic focus.

And in completing the meditation practice:

- reconnecting with the body and senses

- coming back to full waking consciousness

- giving time for feedback.

There are many different meditation techniques, so offering a wide spread of practices means that there will be a method that will work for the individual. Sitting blankly and staring into space is not meditation.

■ Step by step: preparation is everything

Meditation practice can be offered in class and is best placed at the end of the session, after relaxation, when the mind is already in a calmer state. There is a ritual element to meditation that helps to contain and support the practice. If you are at home, you probably have a dedicated place where you can be comfortable and undisturbed. In a classroom situation we have to create a peaceful environment; this may mean helping people to place a blanket or shawl around their shoulders, lowering the lights or lighting a candle. All of this will depend on the space you are using.

A comfortable seated posture is essential, and for most this will be on a chair. An upright spine is helpful even if students have to be propped up. Meditation requires a firm sense of grounding, and in classical practice this is gained by using the lotus position or a comfortable cross-legged posture. Seated, we can achieve a sense of groundedness by feeling into the feet and imagining deep roots growing down, at the same time imagining extending the tail downwards, as if growing a tap root. Breath is the first anchor point to bring balance. Mindful breathing, alternate nostril breathing (Nadi Shodhana Pranyama) can begin the process of developing focus and awareness (see page 222).

Instruction

1. Mudra: Traditionally, the hands are restfully placed on the thighs or knees in Jnana/chin mudra, where the thumb and the tip of the forefinger lightly touch, and the palm can be up (a receptive gesture), or down (for grounding). Alternately, use Dhyana mudra, where the palms are cupped right hand on top of left and the thumbs lightly touching.

2. If neither of these is comfortable, let the hands be placed where they are relaxed, warm and not clenched.

The following are some simple meditation practices that will give grounding for home practice. It is useful to repeat the same practice regularly, as each time the experience will be different.

◼ Dharana: concentration practice

Instruction

1. Focus your attention inwards, and feel as if you are setting aside all of the day's activities and future possibilities. Be present in the 'now'.

2. Begin with some long deep breaths and practise five rounds of alternate nostril breathing (see page 222).

3. Rest the hands using one of the hand (hasta) mudras; this adds to the ritual of the practice, and directs calming energy.

4. Choose a familiar subject for concentration – this is meditation 'with seed'. With this assistance, the mind is given something to do and is less likely to wander.

5. Hold the object in your attention. Notice any time your mind wanders, and gently bring your attention back to the object.

6. After a short time bring your awareness back to noticing your breathing and the feel of your body, and externalise your awareness.

The following could be used as subjects: flowers, candle, fruit, a leaf, pine cone, pebble, sea shell or other natural object, or the focus could be your breathing, or sound.

Teaching focus

- If you are leading meditation, prepare yourself in a similar way to the instructions that you will be giving the class or individual client. If you are calm, grounded and centred, able to focus and steady, you resonate to that calm vibration that facilitates the meditative practice. Students will respond to this.

Parkinson's/MS note: In some people their hands and fingers are badly affected by spasm, and they may not manage a particular mudra. If there is a problem of this type, or an issue with lack of circulation in the hands or feet, make sure that the student will be warm enough – mittens and warm socks may help. Offer a relaxed hand position as an alternative.

Example of a guided concentration practice using an object: Hold the object, or place it where it can be observed closely. Teachers can guide this practice by reminding students of what they are looking at, and how they might lead their thoughts. Using a flower as an object.

Instruction

1. Spend time looking at the flower, taking in all of its details.

2. Notice the colour of the flower. Is it all one colour or is there more than one?

3. Notice the shape of the petals. How many are there? Are they all the same?

4. What is the texture of the petals? Are they soft or stiff, smooth or downy, sticky or prickly?

5. Is the flower fully open? Can you see the centre?

6. What does the centre of the flower look like? What colour is it? How is it formed?

7. Look all around the flower, examine it from underneath, see its shape and form.

8. Is it perfect or windblown? Has it been nibbled by insects?

9. Does it have a scent? What is the scent like?

10. Look at the stem. What is the shape, colour and texture of the stem?

11. Close your eyes and try to hold the image of the flower in your mind's eye. See if you can bring back the memory of the image. If you lose it, look back at the real thing.

12. Take a few moments to think about where the flower grows, what its environment may have been and how it began its life, how it took nutrients from the earth, rain and sun to grow into what you see now. The flower had all of its potential wrapped up in its beginnings. There is a metaphor here for our own growth and development.

Using this questioning enquiry, we can keep the mind engaged on the subject, training focus and concentration. If the mind wanders, bring attention back to the object. This practice can be adjusted in length to fit a time frame available – even ten minutes gives a flavour of a meditation practice, which most will find enjoyable.

So Hum Mantra: using the breath as a focus

This is based on the mantra 'So Hum' ('That I Am'), present in the natural sound of the breath. I find this to be the most useful of all beginners' practices. Not everyone can visualise, but everyone can breathe.

Instruction

1. After preparation, observe the normal flow of breath, without trying to breathe properly.

2. Feel the movement of air in the nostrils, warm and cool.

3. Be aware of where and how the body moves.

4. Be aware of the rhythm of the breathing. Slow it down.

5. Can you find the place where the breath 'starts' down in the abdomen, perhaps? Can you start the breath from lower down?

6. Listen to the natural sound of the breath. In yoga this is described as a mantra. On the inhale the sound is 'so', and on the exhale, 'hum'.

7. Repeat these two sounds mentally as you breathe, 'so' rising up on the inhale, and 'hum' flowing down on the exhale.

8. Take a little time with breathing and repetition of the inner mantra.

9. If your thoughts wander, keep bringing them back to the sound of the breath.

10. It's natural for the mind to wander; just notice when it happens.

11. Gradually increase the time.

This is an excellent and effective practice for students to do by themselves at home, to do if they feel anxious, or to bring a calm state before bedtime.

Teaching focus

- Make a handout of the practice guidelines, as a reminder.
- Allow the students to go at their own pace.
- Remind them that it is normal for the mind to be busy.
- Allow students to keep their eyes open if this helps their balance.

Slowing the thoughts

The following practices offer different ways to understand that thoughts are a function of mind, and that the true self is a separate thing.

Mind clouds

Instruction

1. Prepare and sit comfortably. Steady your breathing, ground and centre.

2. Imagine that you are looking into clear blue sky. Let the blue sky fill your consciousness.

3. As thoughts arise, imagine that they become like fluffy white clouds that drift across the blue sky. As each thought arises, it floats across the sky as a cloud. They may happen in quick succession or more slowly. Some are small wispy clouds and others are big thunder clouds. They all flow across the sky. Look into the spaces between the clouds. Imagine those spaces opening up.

4. The mind is like the sky, and thoughts are like the clouds that float across. We are observing the thoughts, watching them pass across the mind.

5. Gradually become aware that the thoughts are a separate process. You are not your thoughts. They come and go. You, the true self, is watching them.

6. The more practised you become, the more blue sky you see, the thoughts slow down.

■ Pool

Instruction

1. Imagine that you are sitting by a small pond.

2. The surface of the water is still, like a mirror. See the reeds fringing the edge of the pool; notice the plants, the pattern of light and shade, the colours, as you sit quietly.

3. The plants and the sky are reflected in the water. There may be insects hovering over the surface of the water, darting backwards and forwards.

4. As you watch, a bubble floats to the surface; it creates ripples as it breaks. The ripples spread out across the water and melt into the bank. Other bubbles arise and create ripples.

5. These bubbles represent your thoughts – each time a thought occurs, a bubble pops up and disturbs the mirror like surface of the pond.

6. Watch for a little while and be aware of the bubbles. Each time wait for the ripples to stop, until the water becomes a calm clear mirror again.

This image holds within it the philosophy of the mind being a mirror of the true self and that meditation cleans the mirror, so that the true self is revealed.

■ Water lily

Instruction

1. Imagine looking out to see a pool of water; the surface is smooth, the water clear. On the surface floats a water lily.

2. See the flower, its petals delicate and waxy; look closer and see the colour, the petals gently tapering, so fine that you can see the veins running through them.

3. Look to the centre of the flower; see the yellow middle and beneath the flower on the surface of the water imagine the strong green leaf, rounded and leathery.

4. Move back a little and see the petals; the flower looks like a little star floating on the pool. Stay for a moment and hold the image; be aware of what it brings to you – a feeling of peace and stillness, perhaps.

5. Although the flower is delicate, we know that beneath the water are the strong stem and the roots firmly planted in the mud at the bottom of the pool.

The metaphor here is that as we yearn upwards, we need our feet firmly planted on the ground.

■ Seven breaths: becoming calm

This is a simple meditation practice that does not rely on the ability to visualise.

Instruction

1. Sit and be comfortable.

2. Begin to be aware of your breathing.

3. On each exhale count. For example:

   1 – relax

   2 – continue to let go

   3 – release physical tension

   4 – release anxiety

   5 – release fear

   6 – release pain

   7 – become still.

4. Or do your own counting and stay focused. The object is to stay focused; if the mind becomes distracted and you lose count, be aware of what is happening and start again. There is no doing it wrong, just an awareness of what happens.

5. On completing seven breaths, move your attention to the place where the inhale turns into an exhale breath. Pause in that place and bring all your consciousness into that moment.

■ Body scan awareness meditation

Instruction

1. Sit upright. Make sure that you are warm enough and that you are supported in a way that makes you comfortable. Slow down your breathing and let your body relax.

2. Take your attention to your feet. Experience the weight of your feet and the contact that you have with the floor/support. Be aware of any sensations in your feet and how they are feeling – cold, warm, heavy light, tense, soft, etc. Are there any other sensations that you notice, or maybe no sensation?

3. Move your awareness into your ankles; feel around the shape of your bones and observe what you experience in your ankles.

4. Bring your attention into your calves and be aware of how they feel – soft, tight, light, heavy. Any other things that you notice – aches, tingling perhaps? Simply be aware.

5. Move your consciousness into and around your knees. What do you notice here?

6. Now move your awareness into your thighs, the backs of your legs (possibly on a chair), the tops, and be aware of any sensations here.

7. Move your awareness into your 'sit' bones and around your pelvis, feeling the 'sit' bones on the chair and the sensations in and around your pelvis. How do you experience this?

8. Now feel into your middle. What is happening here?

9. Observe without making judgements or evaluating your experience. Let your mind move from one place to another in a dispassionate way – 'I notice this, and now that', and moving on.

10. Move awareness into your upper back, and notice the sensations here. Notice how they begin to change as you place your attention there.

11. Now into your chest; here you can experience your breathing, and the quality and ease of the breath. Is it easy? Tight? Relaxed?

12. Bring awareness into your arms and hands, from the shoulders right down to the tips of your fingers. Be aware of the sensations.

13. Notice any time that your mind wanders, be aware of how that happens and where the mind goes, and then bring your attention back.

14. Feel up into your neck, jaw and head; be aware of the weight of your head, tensions, how you hold your head and anything else you notice.

15. Observe your whole body, your breathing, the stillness. Do not judge yourself or go into any story of why things are this way. Practise a 'detached' observation, so that you are fully aware of what is happening in the present moment.

16. Spend a little time observing this way. Don't try to change it or make it wrong for you to be experiencing this or that, or that you lose focus, or your mind wanders. Let go of criticism.

17. At the end of the practice time, breathe deeply, stretch and become aware of your external surroundings.

◼ Healing meditations

Taking awareness away from the self is in itself a therapeutic practice. The ego becomes smaller and the heart energy grows and radiates, bringing a different perspective on life and love as a way of self-healing. These meditation practices may provoke an emotional response. Allow this, do not stop the flow, keep going, and offer time at the end for the student to be with their feelings. It is important that emotions are not rejected, pushed down or denied. They are part of owning the moment.

◼ Loving kindness meditation: Buddhist origin

Instruction

1. First, find a comfortable position. You can sit or lie down in a position most comfortable for you.

2. Now relax your eyes and close them if you wish. Feel tensions melt away, starting with around your eyes and face, through your neck, shoulders and down your arms. Feel the tension flow away, like a liquid down your body and out through your legs.

3. Feel your body filling up with love. Imagine a loving light entering your feet and legs, up through your body, abdomen, chest and arms.

4. Let that loving feeling focus in your heart, down to your hands and fingers and up to the crown of your head.

5. Feel your body being filled with loving light.

6. Feel it flowing through your body and radiating from your skin.

7. When you feel enveloped in that love, repeat these words:

   – May I be free from all harm. May I be safe and protected.

   – May I be free from all suffering. May I be happy.

   – May I be free from all disease and physical pain. May I be healthy and strong.

   – May I be able to live in this world happily, peacefully, joyfully and with ease.

8. Now think of someone that you hold in esteem. It may be a mentor or a teacher. It can be someone you haven't met but have influenced your life in a positive way. Keeping this person in mind, repeat the statements:

   – May you be free from all harm. May you be safe and protected.

   – May you be free from all suffering. May you be happy.

   – May you be free from all disease and physical pain. May you be healthy and strong.

   – May you be able to live in this world happily, peacefully, joyfully and with ease.

9. Now think of someone that you love dearly. A close family member, lover or friend. Keeping this person in mind, send loving thoughts to him or her. Repeat the following statements:

   – May you be free from all harm. May you be safe and protected.

   – May you be free from all suffering. May you be happy.

   – May you be free from all disease and physical pain. May you be healthy and strong.

   – May you be able to live in this world happily, peacefully, joyfully and with ease.

10. Now think of someone who is an acquaintance, practically a stranger. You do not know this person well. Send loving thoughts to him or her and repeat the following statements:

   – May you be free from all harm. May you be safe and protected.

   – May you be free from all suffering. May you be happy.

   – May you be free from all disease and physical pain. May you be healthy and strong.

   – May you be able to live in this world happily, peacefully, joyfully and with ease.

11. Now think of someone who makes you upset or angry. Still feel the love in your body. Do not let go of this love. Think about this person and send loving thoughts to him or her. Say to them:

   – May you be free from all harm. May you be safe and protected.

   – May you be free from all suffering. May you be happy.

   – May you be free from all disease and physical pain. May you be healthy and strong.

   – May you be able to live in this world happily, peacefully, joyfully and with ease.

12. Now turn your thoughts to this vast world. The earth with all its living creatures. Feel the love bursting through your body as you say:

   – May all beings be free from all harm. May they be safe and protected.

   – May all beings be free from all suffering. May they be happy.

   – May all beings be free from all disease and physical pain. May they be healthy and strong.

   – May all beings be able to live in this world happily, peacefully, joyfully and with ease.

13. Send your love as far out around the world as possible. Imagine that energy travelling through the earth.

14. When you are ready, feel that love centred round your heart.

15. Notice the weight of your feet on the floor or bed. Feel yourself in the now, in the present moment, and when you are ready, open your eyes.

■ Meditation for world peace, with acknowledgment to the Lucis Trust

One of the greatest contributions that we can make to world peace is to find and make peace within ourselves. The more we feel 'upset' about the world situation, or any situation for that matter, the more of the 'upset' vibration we transmit into the world. On a personal health and wellbeing level, upsets are certainly better expressed than suppressed, so the more we can own and acknowledge and find constructive means of expression, the better.

Finding peace in our inner being might be quite a challenge, but also very healing.

Instruction

1. Light a candle dedicated to peace.

2. Sit comfortably, align your spine and steady your breathing.

3. Move your attention to your heart centre.

4. Keep your focus in the heart and be aware of your thoughts and feelings – allow them to flow and observe them.

5. Tune in to where you are right now.

6. Imagine creating a thought of 'perfect peace'; perhaps you have a memory of a time when you felt at peace, even if it was just a short time. Perhaps a memory brings you into peace – a dawn sky, a single rose. Let thoughts and memories around peace settle into your heart.

7. As you touch that thought, allow the feeling of perfect peace to grow, expand and fill your whole being. In this place there is no conflict, no indecision, no resentment. Only benevolence, calm, love, inclusiveness, goodwill.

8. Allow that vibration of peace to radiate from you out into the world.

9. Imagine it flowing to your family and close friends, then out to your neighbours, colleagues, acquaintances (even those you don't like very much). Let it flow out into your community, your town, your county, the country.

10. Let it continue to flow out into the world.

11. See your stream of peace joining others like a network of light around the world.

12. Imagine all your actions and activities coming from the place of perfect peace.

13. Try asking the question 'If I were at peace with myself what would I do, how would I be?' (You might apply this to any situation.)

14. Return to the place of perfect peace within your heart.

15. Remind yourself that it is always there.

16. Resolve to grow the seed of perfect peace in your heart and let it be.

17. Affirm: 'I am in perfect peace.'

18. Move and stretch, go into your day from that place of peace.

Chapter 4

Sample Lesson Plans

These lesson plans are designed to present a simple outline of a typical therapeutic class. A medical history of each student will have been completed before joining the group, so that modifications can be made and individual attention given where necessary. Adjustments, support and modifications are given for each practice.

Sample lesson plan 1

Time: One hour

Support materials: Mat, chair, block. Check the room temperature.

Focus: Overall mobility, strength and stability. Start in a seated position.

Take a moment to get people comfortable; offer a block for under the feet so that good contact can be made. Introduce the plan for the session. This may promote a discussion of personal symptoms or issues.

Encourage an upright spine with natural lumbar curve, sitting on the 'sit' bones. Observe breathing and bring attention into focus ready for yoga. Scan the whole body and identify any trouble spots, discomfort or other experiences. Bring these into focus as the session progresses.

- Neck release: Side turns, up and down movements, and side to side. Aim: to free up the joints and soften the muscles in the upper chest and upper back to enable better breathing.

- Easy shoulder rolls, to ease out shoulder tension. Repeat five times.

- Three-part breath using arm movements. Repeat five times. Aim: to bring awareness of the ribs and back and promote coordination.

Note: Check the students for an upright spine and neck, offer modifications, adjust and support individually.

Safety note: Place a chair within easy reach. Check for contraindications and offer a chair to those unable to stand.

- Mountain Pose (Tadasana). Aim: to bring awareness of posture and alignment.

- Extended Mountain Pose (Tadasana) with core muscles engaged. Lifting and lowering arms, repeat four times.

- Swaying Palm with core muscles engaged.

- Roll forward to rest in Rag Doll Pose, curled spine, released knees, loose head and neck. Check that people are okay standing, and give permission to sit.

- Warrior Pose 1 preparation. Chair to one side, students hold the back of the chair. Aim: to explore stepping and build confidence in placing the feet wider. Take a step forward, check the foot alignment. Engage the pelvic floor. Bend the forward knee. Repeat on the other leg. Check alignment and that students are okay to go further.

- Explore lifting one arm, then both if stable. Ease out any shoulder tension.

- Side bending. Facing the back of the chair, hold with one arm if needed. Do both sides. Counter-pose in a seated position.

- Seated forward bend. Arms lifting, fold forwards and release.

- Feet and ankles, point flex, circle and hold leg extended. Give attention to the standing leg and balance. Aim: to improve mobility and keep good balance.

- Sitting twist. Aim: to free the spinal joints and improve awareness and posture.

- Seated flow. Relaxation. Bring the group to the floor; some may remain seated. Check all supports, head neck, knees, feet.

- Body scan to bring awareness into physical sensations, to energy state, emotional state, observing only a 'snapshot', similarly with the mind. Be aware of our different states of being – body, emotions, mind, energy. Go through the body, part by part, to relax each. Bring awareness to the breath and quiet place of balance in the centre. Bring to full waking consciousness. Ask how the group are doing; stretch and move as you feel. Help the group members to sit up.

If time:

- Sitting: Alternate nostril breathing.

- Short meditation using a flower for focus.

- Namaste.

Sample lesson plan 2

Time: One hour

Support materials: Chair, block, resistance band (varying strengths). Check the room temperature.

Focus: To work the joints.

Start in a seated position. Take a moment to get people comfortable, offer a block for under the feet so that good contact can be made. Introduce the focus for the session, and give time for discussion.

- Encourage an upright spine and sitting on the 'sit' bones.

- Find out how people are today and ask if they have any problems with particular joints. Remind them to only do what they can today. Stop if there is sharp pain.

- Observe breathing and bring attention into focus ready for yoga.

- Sitting: Undulating, Spine, 'C' and 'S' shapes, awareness of any immobile places. Focus on all the spinal joints and free movement.

- Shoulder rolls, alternate movement, backwards and forward. Hands-on guidance for imbalances.

- Standing: Using a resistance band, hold the band between the thumb and hand; discourage clenched fists, arms forward and parallel. Stretch a little wider, feel the action.

- Take the band above the head. Move the left arm down, return and then take the right arm down. Check out any students who are struggling. Repeat two times.

- Bring the band down to thigh level in front of the body, pull it back and release. Repeat four times.

- Full circling movement. Starting above the head, move the arms to the left, and then have the band behind the back. Lift out to the right and up. (This is a useful movement for getting dressed.)

- Hold the chair to assist balance, point, flex and rotate the feet and toes.

- Straight leg with hip rotation.

- *Rest.*

- Move to the mat. Into Cat Pose (Cat/Cow). Core engaged, coordinated breathing.

- Swish the tail: Upper body still, while moving the hips to the left and then right.

- Hip circles. Lift the leg to the side and circle. Make the movement as wide as possible. This helps with getting up and down off the floor.

- Practise bringing the leg through into a kneeling lunge. Rock at the hip.

Relaxation. Bring the group to the floor; some may remain seated. Check all supports, head neck, knees, feet.

- Five kosha awareness. Relaxation to bring balance to all levels.

- Breathe light and golden warmth into every part of the body.

- Bring awareness into the heart. Feel peaceful and quiet.

- Bring to full waking consciousness.

Ask how the group are doing, stretch and move as you feel. Help the group members to sit up.

- Alternate nostril breathing.

- Observe breath, sounds, stillness.

- Namaste.

Sample lesson plan 3

Time: One hour

Support materials: Mat, chair, block and strap. Check the room temperature.
Focus: Working from a chair. To show that a yoga session can be done without getting the mat out if there is restricted space.

Safety: Place the chair on the mat

Start in a seated position on the chair. Discuss home practice, and offer suggestions.

Breath awareness:

- Complete breath, three parts, arms coming out and up. Observe and encourage breathing into the back and sides of the body.

- Sitting in alignment. 'Sit' bones, shoulders, knees, feet. Offer hands-on adjustments to alignment where needed.

- Parallel arms. Breathing with coordination and an up and down arm movement. Watch for the spine staying straight and not arching on lifting.

- Chest-opening breath. Arms opening out to the sides with the breath.

Asana:

- Adapted Cat Pose.

- Leg stretches with foot flex and point. Encourage holding, building strength in the quads. Strong muscles help to avoid joint pain and tendonitis.

- Cycling with one leg at a time. Check for safety and steadiness. Repeat four times on each side.

- Prepare for seated modified Parsvottanasan. Leg straight, supported on a block; reach arms down. Show correct alignment.

- Further the posture by using a strap around the sole of the foot.

- Seated Gate Pose (Parighasana). Explain the benefits and the function of the psoas.

- Simple twist.

Relaxation. Give the group a choice to come to the floor or stay seated. Awareness of the effects of the practice and moving awareness inwards.

- 'So Hum' mantra.

- Stretch gently, move and return to fully awake state.

- Check that everyone is fully present and okay. Invite questions.

- Namaste.

Chapter 5

Class Experiences and Personal Stories

This is a written account of the happenings in our local classes.

Spring 2015: The group work their hips and knees

Today we have Burt, Rose, Sue, Keith, Sheila, James, Bunty, Charlie and Richard. I am supported by Carolyn.

Everyone is fairly mobile and can get up and down off the floor, so we decide to do a floor work session. The room is cool but not cold. Everyone is in reasonable spirits and there is concern among members of the group for Will, who has been taken into hospital with complications after a hip replacement. This group are very close and really look out for each other.

We get everyone down onto the mats with their heads supported, and we begin with slow abdominal breathing, taking it up into full breath, and slowing down the whole thing so that they really arrive and are engaged and centred.

We go on to raising arms with the breath. Some are struggling with shoulder limitations. I encourage them to feel into the back of the ribcage, to keep it down on the mat, and to let the shoulders go within their range without straining.

Moving on to neck roll has my assistant and me checking each person to ensure that necks are straight and that the rotation is aligned.

Shoulder releases follow with lots of enjoyable release as the shoulders drop into the floor.

Now for the real stretching, Charlie has sciatica today, so asks for something to help this specifically. We begin drawing one knee into the chest, encouraging the hip and lower back stretch and holding. We help Keith who can't pull in – a strap around the knee helps him to draw in more effectively. Shirley has had operations on both knees and this is very restricting for her. I carefully add a little pressure to steer and stretch her, asking if it's okay, and going gently.

Directions to circle knees and open up the hip joints are a little more problematic for some, so we give hands-on guidance.

Our next move is to stretch out one leg while the other is held bent. Pushing heels away can cause cramp and some toes are very stiff and reluctant to be turned up. Rose and Sue both have particular issues with spasms in their feet, so we help ease them free, and gradually they respond.

We go on to straightening one leg up to the ceiling; the stretches are gradually getting stronger and everyone is given a strap to help. We assist everyone in keeping their hips level and keeping hips and knees in alignment. Looking around the room, we have various levels of knee angles and hip angles, but we know everyone is working at the hamstring stretch; we encourage them to breathe into the stretch.

We ease out from that into a knees-bent rock. Next up, spinal twist – this should help Charlie's sciatica. We start carefully by asking the group to move both knees only halfway to the left, engage the pelvic floor and keep both shoulders on the mat. We gradually extend this to taking the legs as far as comfortable. Here we can really see how the muscle spasm element of Parkinson's makes the hips and spine stiff. We assist by placing one hand on the shoulder to help it stay put; in some cases we stand behind the student, using our lower leg to support their hips in not rolling back. We give individual attention where it is needed, allowing the group to rest when they are ready before repeating on the other side. This stretch is a real challenge for some people, and yet we know that they welcome the ease and relief that can come after stretching.

We follow this with the same action, but starting by lying on the side, with knees bent. I demonstrate a straight spine aligned with the side of the mat, knees on top of one another, head supported on a block, arms extended in front at shoulder height, palms together. In this asana the arm lifts up to the ceiling, and the turn is centred in the breastbone, rather than the shoulder. We correct arm positions and encourage breastbones to turn rather than arms. They 'get it' and we have a great response, even if the movements are limited, stretching through pectoral muscles and allowing the thoracic spine some movement. This goes a long way in preventing the Parkinson's 'droop'. This is repeated a few times on each side, and again we assist with alignment and encourage pelvic floor and core action to stabilise the lower body.

Next we try keeping the feet together and opening the knees, encouraging the group to engage the core muscles and to squeeze the knees and then the buttocks on opening. There is much good-humoured muttering about this, but everyone gives it a go. Next, a little more action with hip opening and kicking the leg down straight, but in slow motion. More muttering ensues. All of this is, of course, repeated on the other side.

We finish our movements in semi-supine with pelvic tilts moving into Bridge Pose, and finally curled legs and rocking. Everyone is happy at the declaration of relaxation time. We give the group a choice of having a chair to support their legs, sitting on the chair, Corpse Pose (Savasana) or recovery position. We help everyone to find comfort.

This last part of the class is always welcomed. We use a simple awareness-based practice, part by part through the body, beginning with awareness of breath. This week I use a visualisation process that reaches into the memory to imagine the body being strong with confident walking and ease of movement without limitations. We can see that they are engaged with this, by their steadiness, comfort and breathing. Sometimes the tremor will stop. I add in positive affirmations of health and strength.

On completion of the relaxation practice, we gradually arouse people to engage, switch on their senses, starting with sound and moving through touch, sight, taste and smell to connect with the body and the present moment. As people awake, we ask how they are and check that all is well and everyone is fully awake. Sometimes there are questions, but not today. Rose comments on how much she enjoyed all the hip stretches – could we write them down please. Our class ends and we begin to prepare to leave. We always spend time talking to everyone, sharing some of their conversation. Off they go, into the day.

Yoga Therapy group: floor work

Myself and assistant teacher Carolyn, with Keith, Micky (new), Nevil, supported by his son Peter, and Micky's wife Helen, Sue, Sheila, Bunty (supporting James), Joe, Richard and Charlie.

We have a new member today, Nevil, who has arrived with his son to support him; he is quite limited in his transitioning, as is Micky.

I have planned today's class around shoulder and lower back mobility and working on the floor. Nevil shows me his morning stretch that he hopes will help his neck and rounding upper back. This is a typical Parkinson's presentation. The floor will help him to become more aware of alignment and posture and to work his stretching more effectively.

Carolyn and I, with help from the supporters, get the group onto the floor in semi-supine. This takes a little time, as we need to adjust head supports to keep the necks aligned.

We begin by calming the breath, to give people time to adjust and prepare. Neck releasing is the next thing. Some of the group are very experienced in this, which enables us to spend time assisting the newer members, to turn with the head while maintaining a long neck. On to breathing coordination with arm lift. There is a lot to watch for here. We encourage the back of the ribs to stay on the mat, and the shoulders to only go to their limit without straining, We check that each person has 'got' this. Our new member is struggling with his 'messaging' system. This often happens in Parkinson's – people may move their knees instead of their shoulders, for example.

This is followed by shoulder releasing, using the lift and drop action – arms reaching up towards the ceiling and reaching up one arm at a time. We stress the 'let go' part. A small rest now, before moving on to the lower body.

Single knee fold gives another challenge – can they reach and hold the knee? Some cannot, so we offer a strap around the knee. This can lead to over-effort in the struggle to draw the knee close. I show Peter how to help his father, gently guiding the folded knee into the chest to stretch the lower back and to ease out some of the rigidity. Peter agrees to help his father with this at home. Keith is also struggling with this and has a lower back problem, so we assist here too.

Now we work with the twisting action of the spine. With knees together, we get the group to gradually increase their spinal turn movements until they have reached the limit of the spinal twist, and then hold for a few breaths. Again we spend time making sure that shoulders stay on the ground and that people feel into the twisting stretch and possibly even enjoy it! Hands-on assistance is needed for some people – thank goodness we have some family supporters in the room.

A moment of rest to practise abdominal breathing, placing hands over the navel to feel into the breath, and relax with it. We then move on to the pelvic tilt. I really want the students to practise and experience the action of the pelvic floor and abdominal toning, and to be able to ease the lower back and feel some movement here.

We recheck that people are comfortable and aligned. In Parkinson's, people often lose weight, and the bottom of the spine can be a bony place, so a blanket folded and placed under the hips makes a huge difference.

I explain how to press the back of the waist into the floor, and to curl the tail forwards. We bump into the brain messaging problem again, which we commonly meet. We go to each student to check this, placing a hand under the waist and asking the student to press it down. Charlie knows what he wants his body to do, but the message is just not getting through. He applies more focus. I am cheering him on in a quiet way. 'Yes you've got it, keep going, curl up as you breathe out, release and roll the tailbone onto the mat as you breathe in.' He gradually gets there.

And finally we get to relaxation. Going around the body mentally, with awareness. 'Bring in warmth, softness. Let your tensions melt.' I ask them to visualise looking over a farm gate, at a field of ripening wheat. Imagining the wind blowing over the golden wheat and seeing it rippling and waving. 'Lovely warm sunshine, golden wheat waving in the wind.'

Bringing awareness back to full waking consciousness, we get the group moving and stretching. Micky went to sleep, so we gently wake him.

Our new member comes over at the end. 'I really enjoyed that. I could really see that field of wheat waving in the breeze.'

Off they go for their summer break. 'Keep practising and stretching. Have a good summer.'

A restorative session

Two of my more mobile students have come today for an hour's session of restorative practice, something we are unable to do in our regular room as we have no wall space or props. So today we are meeting in my yoga studio, where bolsters, blocks and the like are to hand.

The aim of this session is to see if we can open up the shoulders and allow the spine to let go. We will explore how this may help ease muscle spasm and rigidity, if at all.

I set out mats near the wall, and we begin with some Cat Pose stretches to warm up the spine a little. The first posture is the supported back stretch using one bolster lengthways under the spine.

It takes some time to build the right amount of support with a block under the head and forearms resting on blocks so that the pull on the shoulders is gentle. Both students soon settle into this and are able to hold quite restfully and concentrate on their breathing. They enjoy the openness of the chest, and the stretch through the shoulders; they are able to hold the posture for five minutes or so. They manage to roll out of the posture without too much help from me.

We sit up and move the bolsters in front to support a forward bend; this is harder with only bolsters and blankets, as both students cannot bend so easily. We discuss how this might be done on a chair or by using a large exercise ball.

Next we move to the supported twist. I demonstrate what this will look like and then we position the bolsters. Beryl manages this movement easily, but we have to work a little more with Sheila. As sometimes happens, she is having difficulty with a cramp in her left toe and spasm and stiffness in her left leg, so what would seem like an easy manoeuvre to bring the legs to one side is quite a problem. I help her to shuffle into position enough to lengthen at the front of the body and twist onto the bolster. We get there, and once we are both happy that all is aligned and supported as it should be, both students begin to relax and find the posture comfortable. I encourage them to find the places that are feeling stretched and breathe into them, and also to be aware of the feeling of the twist to the spine.

Coming out of this one is a little easier. Next is the Bound Angle Pose. I demonstrate how we will place the belt, knowing that this will be a challenge. When we have the bolsters in place, belts are added and adjusted. I help them to ease their knees and feet. Heads and necks are supported. This is hard on Sheila – her feet are uncomfortable even supported on a soft foam block, so it's not going to work for her today. I explain that we do not need to struggle, that it is meant to be restful and relaxing. Beryl has more success. I prop up her knees and thighs, and we get the stretch through the groin and adductors, and then cramp sets into her calves, so we ease her out gently.

Lastly Legs-up-the-Wall Pose (Viparita Karani). We use two mats to provide more comfort for bony spines, and I show them how to get into position. This is not easy when your body does not quite move in the way you want it. So mats side by side give rolling room. Eventually, both get there, not quite as upright as it would look 'in the book', but legs are elevated and blocks in place to lift the hips. Success! We lift a little higher onto the bolsters. Both declare this good. Rolling out carefully, we discuss how this might work at home, and before we know it, our hour is over.

Personal stories

Sylvia has been diagnosed with Parkinson's since she was in her forties, and 20 years later, she is still mobile and active, although not without problems. She has been attending a yoga class especially for people with Parkinson's since its inception, 15 years ago. She has knee problems now, and although she has had treatment for both, this has limited her movements considerably. Rigidity and muscle spasm blight her feet and toes, and restrict her upper back. She remains positive and adapts postures for herself; she uses cushions to aid her comfort in relaxation, but will always attempt the standing postures, even when her balance is not good. She has a tremendously positive attitude and is a real fighter. She does some kind of exercise every day, and would sign up for a yoga class every day, as for her it has been the most useful of all the supportive activities on offer in her locality. This same view is held by her husband, who sees a big difference in Sylvia when she has been practising yoga.

Pam came to see me a few summers ago. She was in the early stages of her diagnosis and still coming to terms with the 'label', and it was important for her to appear and be 'normal' although her movements were slowing, her physical symptoms were not too severe, but her anxiety high. She was going to Tai Chi and was reluctant to join a class especially for people with Parkinson's. Many people find that the prospect of this is a frightening thing, an admission that the disease is present, and therefore to go to a 'special' class would be giving in to it. Many are frightened of seeing others who may be further on in the disease process and can't cope with the idea that this may be a probability for them, even though each individual is different and the progress is different. For Pam, her main concern was that her toes were 'not working'. When your feet are numb and you can't feel them properly, your ability to walk, balance and trust in the ground in shaken. We spent three sessions 'feeling' into the feet, 'inking' the soles, putting roots down and anchoring into the ground. We added working the toes and ankles, putting them through their paces, and practising some balances to activate proprioception. Pam was diligent in practising daily, and after three weeks reported a big difference in her foot mobility. She reported that her feet were more responsive and less rigid.

Jane came to class with her husband. She had been diagnosed with Parkinson's and had attended regular yoga classes in the past. Her husband, Ronald, was quite ill, suffering from an undiagnosed lung problem that left him very short of breath. Jane was obviously under a lot of stress and had hoped that yoga would help his breathing. Ronald's consultant had agreed that yoga might be the best thing to help him. Her initial attendance had been as much for his benefit as for hers. Jane found that for her yoga was greatly helpful, particularly the breathing and the relaxation practices, helping her through a very stressful time. Although her husband did find that he felt better and could breathe more easily with yoga practice, sadly his condition worsened and cancer was diagnosed. Jane was left widowed and alone to manage her Parkinson's. Jane has continued to come to class and is finding that her arm swing is returning; this was one symptom that was very noticeable for her. This improvement has given her confidence and has boosted her determination to continue to move, stretch and mobilise.

Katherine has recently chosen to go for deep brain stimulation surgery after her 'off' periods were becoming more of a problem, with trembling and involuntary movements impeding her quality of life. Katherine finds that the stretches and awareness of balance and posture have helped her greatly. At her recent hospital evaluation for her surgery, the health professionals were able to see the improvements in balance and alignment that yoga and Conductive Education had made, and commented on the benefits. Many of the benefits that yoga brings are noted by other health professionals.

Wendy arranged to do some one-to-one yoga sessions to see if they would help keep her moving and build some strength. With a busy, stressful business to run, her time for attending a class was limited, and, like many with MS, she would run out of steam before evening, so a daytime session suited her better. Tight neck and shoulders and sluggish digestion were our main focus at first. Fiercely independent and a hard worker, switching off was of prime importance, and it gradually became clear that deep relaxation was of great benefit and provided supportive switch-off time. Her practice included Pranayama, and upper body stretches to release the shoulders head and neck, simple Wind-Relieving Pose (Pawanmuktasana), and shoulder drop releases, Warrior and balancing for building stability, and supine and seated twists to provide a deep massage for the digestive tract.

Wendy used sessions of colonic irrigation to help her digestive system, and her therapist would always know if she had been neglecting her yoga practice, showing that the outer actions have a real effect on the inner workings. On being asked, 'What is the most helpful of all the yoga practices?', relaxation came top of her list.

I began to work with yoga for improvement of health and wellbeing in someone with Parkinson's sometime in the 1980s. I was experimenting with dowsing to ascertain levels of energy in the chakras, and giving a talk to a group and demonstrating what the dowsing would reveal. I asked for a volunteer. A lady stepped forward and I proceeded to go through the dowsing technique. Starting with base chakra, the result was low static energy – 'a problem', I thought, saying nothing. Other centres were average until I got to the brow and crown – again, not much energy or flow. There is something serious going on here, I thought. I then asked if the lady had any health problems. 'I have Parkinson's disease,' she said.

Although I did not understand and could not have diagnosed my own reading at that time, now it makes perfect sense. I began to work with this lady on a weekly basis. Her breathing improved and she practised daily; her balance improved and she stayed active. Life moved on and I moved away. But I will always remember that chakra reading showing up the physical disturbance in the brain and in the action of walking, and in the inability for the brain to communicate with the body, evident in the readings of the crown and the base. It started me on a long journey.

Resources

For information on all aspects of Parkinson's disease:

American Parkinson Disease Association (APDA), 135 Parkinson Avenue, Staten Island, NY 10305, USA.
Tel. 800-223-2732 or 718-981-8001
www.apdaparkinson.org

National Parkinson Foundation, 200 SE 1st Street, Suite 800, Miami, Florida 33131, USA.
Toll-free Helpline: 1-800-4PD-INFO (473-4636)
www.parkinson.org

Parkinson's UK, 215 Vauxhall Bridge Road, London SW1V 1EJ.
Tel. 020 7931 8080
www.parkinsons.org.uk

For information on all aspects of multiple sclerosis:

Multiple Sclerosis Association of America (MSAA), National Headquarters, 375 Kings Highway North, Cherry Hill, NJ 08034, USA.
Tel. (800) 532-7667
http://mymsaa.org

Multiple Sclerosis (MS) Society, MS National Centre (MSNC), 372 Edgware Road, London NW2 6ND.
Tel. 020 8438 0700
www.mssociety.org.uk/contact-us

Multiple Sclerosis (MS) Trust, Spirella Building, Bridge Road, Letchworth Garden City, Hertfordshire SG6 4ET.
Tel. 0800 032 3839
www.mstrust.org.uk

Yoga Therapy:

British Council for Yoga Therapy (BCYT)
www.bcyt.co.uk

The International Association of Yoga Therapists (IAYT)
Tel. 928-541-0004
www.iayt.org

References

Blashki, H. (2008) Presentation from a minor thesis for the Graduate Certificate in Yoga Therapy, Australian tertiary accredited course code 21720VIC. Melbourne, Australia.

Boser, A. (2007) *Relieve Stiffness and Feel Young Again with Undulation.* Issaquah, WA: Vital Self.

Boulgarides, L., Coleman Salgado, B., Barakatt, E., Choo, D., El-Zahr, M., Williams, K. and Morales, A. (2008) *Effect of an Eight-week Adaptive Yoga Program on Mobility, Function, and Outlook in Individuals with Parkinson's Disease.* Sacramento State. Available at Available at http://c.ymcdn.com/sites/www.iayt.org/resource/resmgr/DRL_Attachments/SYTAR5Mar08.pdf, accessed on 16 March 2016.

Charmaz, K. (1983) 'Loss of self: A fundamental form of suffering in the chronically ill.' *Sociology of Health and Illness 5*, 2. Available at http://qmplus.qmul.ac.uk/pluginfile.php/158532/mod_book/chapter/3334/Charmaz%20K.pdf, accessed on 16 March 2016.

Desikachar, T.K.V. (1999) *The Heart of Yoga: Developing a Personal Practice.* Rochester, VT: Inner Traditions International.

Doherty, K.M., Davagnanam, I., Molloy, S., Silveira-Morlyama, L. and Lees, A.J. (2013) 'Pisa syndrome in Parkinson's disease: A mobile or fixed deformity?' *Journal of Neurology, Neurosurgery and Psychiatry.* doi:10.1136/jnnp-2012-304700. See more at www.parkinsons.org.uk/content/why-do-people-parkinsons-have-difficulty-posture

Fogerite, S.G., Cohen, E., Kietrys, D., Silva, M., Speer, D., Ahrens, S. *et al.* (2014) 'Pilot trial of an integrative yoga program designed by a Delphi method for people with moderate disability due to Multiple Sclerosis.' *The Journal of Alternative and Complementary Medicine 20*, 5, A22–A22. Available at http://online.liebertpub.com/doi/abs/10.1089/acm.2014.5054.abstract, accessed on 10 May 2016. See also http://news.rutgers.edu/feature/yoga-relieves-multiple-sclerosis-symptoms-rutgers-study-finds/20140901#.VzHDG2bBcot

Gallwey, W.T. (1975) *The Inner Game of Tennis: The Ultimate Guide to the Mental Side of Peak Performance.* London: Pan Books.

Goyal, M., Singh, S., Sibinga, E.M.S., Gould, N.F., Rowland-Seymour, A., Sharma, R. *et al.* (2014) 'Meditation programs for psychological stress: A systematic review and meta-analysis.' *JAMA Internal Medicine 174*, 3, 357–368. See also www.sciencedaily.com/releases/2014/01/140106190050.htm

Hoehn, M.M. and Yahr, M.D. (1967) 'Parkinsonism: Onset, progression, and mortality.' *Neurology 17*, 427–442. Available at www.neurology.org/content/17/5/427.full.pdf, accessed on 16 March 2016.

Hogan, G. (2009) *A Relationship with the Chakras: Alleviating Pain in Our Bodies.* Melbourne, Australia: Australian Institute of Yoga Therapy and the Centre for Adult Education, under the supervision of Dr Angela Hass.

Kigi, K.A. *et al.* (2005) 'Intracerebral pain processing in a yoga master who claims not to feel pain during meditation.' National Centre for Biotechnology Information.

Lasater, J.H. (2011) *Relax and Renew: Restful Yoga for Stressful* Times. Berkeley, CA: Rodmell Press.

Lucis Trust, www.lucistrust.org/world_goodwill, London, New York, Geneva.

McGonigal, K. (2009) *Yoga for Pain Relief: Simple Practices to Calm Your Mind and Heal Your Chronic Pain.* Oakland, CA: New Harbinger Publications.

Melzack, R. and Wall, P.D. (1965) 'Pain mechanisms: a new theory.' *Science 150,* 971–979.

Multiple Sclerosis (MS) Society (no date) Available at www.mssociety.org.uk/search/apachesolr_search/diet%20and%20MS, accessed on 9 May 2016.

Multiple Sclerosis (MS) Trust (2014) *Diet.* Available at https://www.mstrust.org.uk/a-z/diet, accessed on 11 July 2016.

NHS Choices (no date) 'Living with pain.' Available at www.nhs.uk/Livewell/Pain/Pages/Painhome.aspx, accessed on 15 March 2016.

Osborn, M. and Rodham, K. (2010) 'Insights into pain: A review of qualitative research.' *British Journal of Pain 4,* 1, 2–7.

Parkinson's UK (no date) 'Deep brain stimulation surgery for Parkinson's.' Available at www.parkinsons.org.uk/content/deep-brain-stimulation-surgery-parkinsons, accessed on 9 May 2016.

Parkinson's UK (no date) 'Parkinson's medication, diet and supplements.' Available at www.parkinsons.org.uk/content/parkinsons-medication-diet-and-supplements, accessed on 9 May 2016.

Pert, C.B. (1999) *Molecules of Emotion: Why You Feel the Way You Feel.* London: Pocket Books.

Porges, S.W. (2011) 'The polyvagal theory: New insights into adaptive reactions of the autonomic nervous system.' *Cleveland Clinic Journal of Medicine 76,* 2, S86–S90.

Roland, K.P, Cornett K.M.D., Theou, O., Jakobi, J.M. and Jones, G.R. (2005) 'Physical Activity across Frailty Phenotypes in Females with Parkinson's Disease.' University of British Columbia.

Rubenstein, L. and Roseman, T. (2011) 'Neuroplastic Yoga for Chronic Pain.' Lecture at International Association of Yoga Teachers (IAYT) conference.

Satchidananda, S.S. (2012) *The Yoga Sutras of Patanjali.* Buckingham, VA: Integral Yoga® Publications.

The Expanding Light (2008) *Yoga Postures and Meditation for Persons with Multiple Sclerosis.* Nevada City, CA: The Expanding Light Meditation and Yoga Retreat.

Index